Measurement and Analysis in Transforming Healthcare Delivery

Peter J. Fabri

Measurement and Analysis in Transforming Healthcare Delivery

Volume 1: Quantitative Approaches in Health Systems Engineering

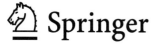 Springer

Peter J. Fabri
Colleges of Medicine and Engineering
University of South Florida
Tampa, FL, USA

ISBN 978-3-319-82190-0   ISBN 978-3-319-40812-5   (eBook)
DOI 10.1007/978-3-319-40812-5

Printed on acid-free paper

This Springer imprint is published by Springer Nature
The registered company is Springer International Publishing AG Switzerland

To my loving wife, Sharon, who put up with me through the struggles of returning to graduate school, who actually understood why a successful academic surgeon would start all over in order to develop a new approach to "fixing healthcare," and who encouraged me to write this book. To my children, Christopher and Andrea, who still think I'm crazy. To Tony Dorfmueller, who introduced me to Total Quality Management and Continuous Quality Improvement long before these concepts were recognized in healthcare. To Thomas Graf MD who provided expert feedback. To Louis Martin-Vega PhD and Jose Zayas-Castro PhD who believed in me and allowed me to pursue a PhD in Industrial Engineering 36 years after I completed college and without any prior education in engineering [3]. And to my students, both in medicine and in engineering, who helped me formulate new ways to explain difficult analytical and quantitative concepts.

Preface

In general, one might conclude that relatively too much scientific effort has been expended hitherto in the production of new devices and too little in the proper use of what we have got.

Patrick Maynard Stuart Blackett, Baron Blackett OM CH PRS [1]

In the opening salvos of the Second World War, Britain, which fully believed in its own superiority and prowess, found itself totally stymied by the creative attacks of the Germans by sea and by air. A group of British scientists, armed primarily with knowledge of probability, statistics, and the ability to analyze and understand data, and using existing technology, developed new methods of implementation which dramatically increased effectiveness and turned the tide of the war. This new field (called operations research, which later evolved into Systems Engineering) TRANSFORMED how the military engaged in war. This book is intended to stimulate and encourage like-minded physicians to use measurement and analysis of existing "operations" to implement new strategic approaches to transform healthcare delivery [2].

About 15 years ago, after over 3 decades as an academic physician, most of them in leadership and management positions, I reached the conclusion that the problems with US healthcare were NOT management and finance problems but rather system and process problems. This was in stark contrast to the traditional belief that the solution to healthcare for a physician was to get an executive MBA. The Institute of Medicine had recently published "To Err Is Human," in which they convincingly demonstrated that US healthcare was manifestly unsafe, and "Crossing the Quality Chasm," in which they laid out the six goals for quality in healthcare: safe, effective, patient centered, timely, efficient, equitable (SEPTEE). I had recently been asked to serve on the thesis committee for a graduate student in the Department of Industrial and Management Systems Engineering. I had previously served on a number of thesis and dissertation committees in other colleges and departments, presumably because I could serve as a link between the underlying basic discipline and the healthcare world. In this case, the graduate student wanted to determine if reengineering could be applied to graduate medical education and I was the Associate

Dean for GME. This adventure opened my eyes to the possibility that formal industrial engineering concepts could be adapted and applied to healthcare. Shortly after, I was asked to co-chair a committee to create a new joint degree program (MD-PhD) in biomedical engineering, which put me in close contact with the Dean of the College of Engineering. One day, I suggested to him that he needed a "stalking horse" to go through the engineering program and offered to be that person. To my surprise, he responded that if I could meet the admission requirements, I was in. More surprisingly, the rest is history.

When I completed my PhD in Industrial Engineering, already a tenured full professor in the College of Medicine, I was eligible for a sabbatical. I was given the opportunity to spend a semester at Northwestern University, with highly regarded colleges of Medicine and Engineering that were physically separated by a dozen difficult Chicago miles, allowing me to introduce a "bridge" between two entities that while part of the same university were geographically and culturally separate. More importantly, Chicago served as the headquarters of nearly every major medical organization and association. With these "collaborators," I set out to develop a needs assessment and a curriculum for a graduate degree program in Health Systems Engineering. Returning to the University of South Florida, I was asked to teach an engineering course in Linear Programming and Operations Research. I embraced this as an opportunity to begin to meld the medical approach to learning and understanding with the rigorous mathematics and computer science of Industrial Engineering. I was subsequently asked to create a new course in Engineering Analytics. And again, the rest is history.

Over the ensuing years, I was asked to teach other fundamental engineering courses, while each time looking for ways to "reinterpret" the material in ways acceptable and understandable to physicians and other clinicians. This background allowed me to develop and institute a "Scholarly Concentration" within the medical school entitled Health Systems Engineering, which included four 1-year courses taught concurrently with the medical school curriculum: Human Error and Patient Safety; Systems Modeling and Optimization; Data Mining and Analytics; and Quality Management, LEAN, Six Sigma. As of this date, over 50 medical students have enrolled in this program, with only a handful having prior education in engineering. Based on their experiences, several of these medical students elected to pursue advanced degrees in engineering while in medical school, one without having had any prior engineering education.

With these prototypes in the Colleges of Medicine and Engineering, I approached the American College of Surgeons with the idea of creating a program in Health Systems Engineering for practicing surgeons. Surprisingly, they embraced the concept and we created a series of postgraduate courses, DVDs, and educational curricula in Health Systems Engineering specifically for surgeons.

Based on these endeavors, I now propose a textbook whose purpose is to present difficult analytical concepts and approaches to motivated physicians who are willing to embrace the challenge of creating a "toolbox" to help them fix healthcare. This toolbox includes new ways to approach quality and safety, new understanding of data analysis and statistics, and new tools to analyze and understand healthcare delivery and how it can be improved. All of this is predicated on the well-accepted engineering principle—if you can't measure it, you can't improve it.

The intent of this book is NOT to turn physicians into engineers. Rather, it is to create physicians who are "bilingual," who can speak the language of statistics and systems engineering, and who can become active participants in the transformation of healthcare.

Tampa, FL, USA   Peter J. Fabri

References

1. Blackett PMS. Scientists at the operational level, notes on statement to Admiralty Panel on 9/16/1941 on the function of the operational research station. Blackett Papers, PB 4/7/1/2.
2. Budiansky S. Blackett's war. 1st ed. New York: Alfred A. Knopf; 2013. 306p.
3. Fabri PJ, Zayas-Castro JL. Human error, not communication and systems, underlies surgical complications. Surgery. 2008;144(4):557–63; discussion 63–5.

Contents

Chapter 1
Introduction to Measurement and Analysis

Scenario

Dr. Ben Griffin has just been asked by the CEO of East Coast Medical Center to chair a group to help position the hospital for success under the Accountable Care Act. Ben is a very successful cardiac surgeon who is highly respected because of the volume of his clinical practice and his leadership skills. At the first meeting of the group, he is introduced to the team: a systems analyst, a biostatistician, an accountant, a nurse manager, and the director of research. He immediately realizes that he doesn't even speak the same language that they are using. And they're not looking for a "captain"; they're looking for a clinical colleague. Not wanting to be embarrassed or to let the CEO down, Ben commits himself to learning more about what these people know how to do and how they look at the problem **(machine learning; supervised and unsupervised learning)**.

1.1 Key Questions Regarding Health Systems Engineering

Consider this text as a "primer" on fixing healthcare. That statement should provoke a series of questions.

1.1.1 What's Wrong with Healthcare?

Healthcare, at least as we know it, really developed in the 1950s and 1960s, when physicians were in solo, private practice, few patients had health insurance, Medicare hadn't been invented, and patients often came to the office with chickens in hand to

© Springer International Publishing Switzerland 2016
P.J. Fabri, *Measurement and Analysis in Transforming Healthcare Delivery*,
DOI 10.1007/978-3-319-40812-5_1

pay for their visit. Computers only existed in large universities (and then usually only one!); transistors hadn't worked their way into manufacturing; diodes and silicon chips were years away. As for communication, you had to speak to the operator to make a telephone call on a party line phone shared with several neighbors. Medications were administered either by mouth or intramuscularly and IV meds, either "push" or infusion, weren't commonly used. There were no ICUs, transplants, dialysis, or heart surgery. In short, most of what we take for granted today didn't exist. The subsequent tsunami of technology and science developments has overwhelmed our ability to fully comprehend them, let alone master them. Consider, for example, a smart phone. How much of the capability of this ubiquitous device do you actually understand? How much can you actually use? Yet you walk around with it in your pocket every day. No, we never actually learned HOW TO USE CORRECTLY many of the things we take for granted.

You have probably heard the terms "systems" and "processes." You may even have adopted them into your vocabulary. What do they mean? **A system is a set of interrelated activities that lead to a <u>common goal</u>. A process is a set of interconnected steps that result in a <u>product or outcome</u>** [1]. More importantly, these terms imply "standardization." If "<u>I</u>" have a system for preparing myself to go to work in the morning, would <u>"you"</u> agree that it is a system? No, you have your way and I have my way, and you probably think my way doesn't make much sense. The same is true in healthcare. Our "systems" are very local rule sets that typically aren't shared by anybody else. They are "haphazard systems" or "non-systems." So in this complex, multimedia-driven, interconnected world of healthcare, our sets of "systems" often clash. What makes this an untenable situation is that virtually every other aspect of our lives—banking, airline travel, and checking out at the grocery store—has moved ahead, developing functioning integrated systems and processes, while we are still functioning the way doctors' offices functioned in the 1950s and 1960s.

Did you take a course in medical school to prepare you for practice? Perhaps (if you were lucky) you learned a bit about billing and scheduling, but probably not. Did you learn about optimization? Metrics? Safety? Outcome analysis? Continuous quality improvement? LEAN? Six-Sigma? Statistical process control? No, very few physicians were introduced to any of these concepts, nor were they usually picked up "along the way." In commerce and industry an organization that didn't learn these concepts has gone the way of the dinosaur. In healthcare, it's still the rule.

In college, did you learn enough advanced mathematics, logic, and computer science to be able to develop analytical models of your practice outcomes? Or to conduct a thorough evaluation of why an operation or procedure didn't work out the way it was intended?

In summary, in medical school we learned about medicine. Even in residency, we only learned about medicine. Physicians have largely been "hands off" regarding quality and safety, and the consequence is that if anybody has been driving this "battleship," it wasn't us. But it appears that, for the most part, nobody else was at the wheel either!

1.1.2   Why Should "I" Fix It?

As I often tell my students, "if you wait until it gets fixed by lawyers and politicians, don't get upset if it looks like it was fixed by lawyers and politicians." In other words, the only people who can "intelligently" fix how US healthcare is implemented, conducted, analyzed, modified, and perceived are PHYSICIANS WHO ARE PREPARED to fix it.

You might respond that you are not an engineer or even a computer scientist. But as I tell the first-year medical students during a presentation about the Health Systems Engineering Scholarly Concentration, they don't need to be engineers. They only need to have LIKED math and physics in college. They didn't even have to be good at it. They only had to LIKE it. That plus the motivation to actually want to make a major contribution to the future of US healthcare is all that is required. Plus a little patience and diligence, of course, and a fair amount of work.

It would be over-simplistic to say that learning about advanced mathematics, graphics, computers, and statistics is easy. It isn't. But it's absolutely possible, particularly if the material is explained in a way that makes sense to a physician. Hopefully, this text will resonate with how you have learned and how you have thought while at the same time stimulating you to learn to think in new ways. The purpose of this book is NOT to create engineers. It is to create physicians who are "bilingual."

1.1.3   What Is Health Systems Engineering?

Although there are certainly examples of industrial engineering concepts prior to World War II, it was really that war, with all of the complexities of a truly global war in two major theaters, which led to the development of modern systems engineering [2]. Although computers as we know them were still at least a decade in the future, methods were already being developed for optimizing, analyzing, and interpreting complex operations. From this nucleus, the field of industrial and systems engineering developed. At the same time, in post-war Japan, the concepts of continuous quality improvement were being developed by W. Edwards Deming and Joseph Juran [3]. Although Juran made a major contribution, the concepts of total quality management (TQM) and continuous quality improvement (CQI) in healthcare are usually credited to Deming [4]. The third piece in this puzzle didn't emerge until the mid-1970s to mid-1980s as the result of three disastrous events: the Tenerife aircraft disaster (1977), the Three Mile Island nuclear power plant meltdown in Pennsylvania (1979), and the Chernobyl nuclear power plant explosion (1986) [5]. These three events are generally credited for refocusing the development of human error analysis from its origins in cognitive psychology. While not an "all-inclusive" list, for our purposes systems engineering, quality management and improvement, and human error and patient safety form the springboard for the development of health systems engineering (HSE). HSE, then, is the adaptation and application of tools and methods developed in these key areas to the domain of healthcare. It is very important to reiterate that the focus is NOT management and finance. The key concept is that focusing on quality and safety LEADS to economic benefit. This lesson has been learned through the US industry over the past 40 years, albeit slowly and with many "hiccups" [6]. The corollary lesson learned is that organizations that fail to shift their commitment to quality regularly "fail." To date, the lessons learned in industry, and we're talking first "hard" industry (rubber, coal, steel), then soft industry (computers, manufacturing), and finally service industry (aviation, telephones, Internet, etc.), have gone unheeded in healthcare. The auto industry strongly resisted, and all of the Big Three faced bankruptcy during the last decade! Only in the past 5 years have they refocused on quality with dramatic impact on their bottom line. What is the likely attitude in healthcare?

It is extremely likely that barring some major cataclysm, the same fundamental, status-quo principles will continue to drive the next decade of healthcare delivery. Until now, healthcare (hospitals, providers, pharmaceuticals, etc.) has been able to name its own price and it would be paid. There was no "incentive" to focus on quality. But the newly minted accountable care organizations will require high quality, efficiency, and safety. Individuals and organizations that are "prepared to make a difference" will be well positioned in this new world of healthcare [7].

1.1.4   What Is "Analytics"?

Analytics is a term and a concept which has developed over the past 5–10 years, built on a solid 100-year tradition of statistics [8]. The driving force for the development of analytics has been the emergence of large databases, collected for a variety of reasons over the past 20–40 years, and the desire to try to understand what is in them and to use that knowledge to develop models to understand what happened and to predict what is going to happen next. If we studied statistics, either in college or in medical school/professional school, we would have studied "parametric statistics," which is based on the concept of the bell-shaped curve and its application to designed experiments. The data generated from designed experiments are "neat," "orderly," and "systematic," and the statistical approach is determined PRIOR to collecting the data. The hypothesis is clear and unambiguous. Databases and data collected in the process of doing things are a very different animal with many limitations and quirks. The data were collected for a different purpose; the included variables were selected to address a different need; a large number of other alternate hypotheses (not just one alternate) are possible. The medical literature is progressively including more and more articles about outcomes, safety, quality, and the like, but the statistics are typically the same statistics that are used in a designed experiment, without attention to the limitations and quirks. Analytics attempts to introduce a different approach to applying the same fundamental statistical concepts in ways that more appropriately "fit." A large part of this difference is in understanding, "polishing," and visualizing the data. Another large part is applying methods that will address the serious limitations and quirks that a traditional statistical approach engenders.

1.1.5   Is This an Individual Activity or an Organizational Activity?

While individual effort will certainly be necessary (which will require individuals who are PREPARED TO MAKE A DIFFERENCE), quality and safety ultimately involve organizations. This will necessitate improved communication, development of standardized approaches, sharing data, teamwork, shared responsibility, and, perhaps most importantly, a shared vision and a supportive culture. None of these are currently part of the "fiber" of US healthcare, so they will need to be developed, nurtured, and led [9]. Since physicians play an instrumental role in the leadership of healthcare delivery organizations, and since physicians ultimately have the most to gain or lose from success (other than the patients, of course!), it is critical that individual physicians develop the knowledge, technical skills, and behavioral skills (the competencies of quality and safety) necessary to lead in the development of shared visions and a supportive culture [9].

1.2   The Organization of This Book

Since much of the material covered in this text is genuinely "new" material for physicians, it will build from background through fundamentals into application. The end result should be a set of competencies (knowledge, technical skills, and behavioral skills) that will allow the physician/practitioner to participate in the process of transforming healthcare locally, regionally, and even nationally.

There are four parts to this book: **Managing Data, Applying a Scientific Approach to Data Analysis, Methods to Analyze Data, and Interpreting Outcomes and Anticipating Failures**. Underlying each of these is the fundamental concept that in order to improve something, outcomes must be measured in a reliable (repeatable) and valid (accurate) way. Part 1, **Managing Data**, will go back to mathematical fundamentals regarding measurement and uncertainty. In order to make this practical, we will begin to learn about readily available **computer software** to help us manage and analyze the data. We will begin to think about each individual "number" or "fact" as having an element of uncertainty, known as **stochastic** (subject to random variability). We will address "**error**" (both random and systematic) and how to deal with it as well as "missing values." We will then reinterpret columns of data and rows of subjects/patients as sets of numbers known as **vectors**. We will consider not only the "normal" distribution, but also other common **distributions** that occur in the medical domain. We will begin to use and understand data by addressing advanced skills in Microsoft Excel, and we will consider additional software tools to allow us to do computer **modeling** and interpretation. We will start using graphs and charts to **visualize** data. Once we have a reasonable grasp of what data ARE and how to use THEM, we will address the application of the **scientific method** in **retrospective analysis** to better understand and interpret the underlying meanings of the data. The first section also introduces advanced analytical capabilities of Microsoft Excel. This section presumes that you have a fundamental understanding of Excel (how to use a spreadsheet, how to enter data, how to perform row and column operations) and focuses on visualization and data analysis tools that can be useful in the preliminary assessment of data.

Part 2, **Applying a Scientific Approach to Data Analysis**, addresses the fundamental aspects of understanding data at a deeper level and of being able to apply mathematical and statistical concepts. Woven throughout Part 2 is the concept of **distributions of data**, which are often best assessed by **visualization** using graphs and histograms. The **normal distribution** (bell-shaped curve or Gaussian distribution) is discussed first, because it is the traditional method taught in college classes of statistics, followed by other important distributions useful in clinical medicine. We then discuss the "problem areas" in dealing with data, particularly too many variables (**dimensionality**, **over- and under-fitting**), highly correlated variables (**multicollinearity**), small sample size, and **nonhomogeneous** datasets (**heteroscedasticity**). Finally we address basic but relevant concepts of probability, how they are important in understanding data, and how they relate to statistics and the application of statistical methods.

Part 3, **Methods to Analyze Data**, gets into the nitty-gritty number crunching necessary to make sense of complex data. It starts with a discussion of models (a **model** is a replica or representation of reality, usually in simplified form), **modeling** (the process of building or creating a model), and **predictive models** (mathematical constructs that predict an outcome from a set of input variables). It addresses the application of statistical methods and model building to computer analysis of data, known as **machine learning**. It clarifies the difference between modeling data when an outcome is given (known as **supervised learning** because you can actually validate the model against a known outcome), and when either there is no outcome, just data or when you choose to overlook the outcome in model building (**unsupervised learning**). The two major dimensions of supervised model building, **regression** and **classification**, are presented, including the major methods currently used in the medical and scientific literature for accomplishing them. Regression is the term that describes predictive model building when the outcome variable is continuous. Classification is exactly analogous except that the outcome variable is categorical (usually binary, yes-no). We will go well beyond the traditional methods of **multiple regression** (single continuous outcome with multiple input variables) and logistic regression (single binary outcome with multiple input variables) because of the frequent need to address some important "flaw" in the data, such as dimensionality, collinearity, and non-homogeneity, describing modern methods that were created specifically to address these limitations or violations of assumptions.

We then address data analysis in the absence of an outcome variable, **unsupervised learning**. Such situations usually occur in two situations, qualitative "lists," often referred to as **market-baskets**, and quantitative spreadsheets with attributes but not outcomes. In the market-basket scenario, since what might appear as "data" is really a set of **nominal attributes**, formal analysis is limited to counting and describing lists, referred to as **association analysis**. Further mathematical and statistical analysis is not possible when the data are nominal. When the variables are quantitative (continuous) but in the absence of an outcome variable, various techniques of **clustering** can be applied, using defined measures of **proximity, distance,** or **similarity**. Clustering can also be used in situations when an outcome variable actually exists but is set aside temporarily to better define and understand the structure of the data, prior to applying supervised methods.

Often medical analysis addresses measures over time, which requires methods based on concepts of survival. **Survival methods** are based on a concept known as the **survival function**, which is just 1 minus a failure rate. It can most easily be thought of as what percentage of individuals are still alive (or the inverse, who died) GIVEN the number who were alive at the beginning of the time interval (such as a year). A **hazard function** is then defined as a mathematical derivation of the survival function – minus the slope of the logarithm of the survival function ($-d(\log S)/dt$). This allows calculation of what are known as **actuarial survival curves** using the methodology of Kaplan-Meier, and comparing survival curves using the **log-rank test**. When analysis of survival includes addressing input variables that might affect survival, we perform a **Cox proportional hazard analysis**.

Closing Part 3, we also look at the **assumptions** inherent in each of these modeling approaches, so as to know when the models/methods are not applicable or at least require modifications in interpretation.

Part 4, **Interpreting Outcomes and Anticipating Failures,** first introduces the application and limitation of interpretation of results, and addresses a number of concepts that are frequently misunderstood or overlooked in medical analytics, specifically "cause and effect." **Outliers** are considered next and represent results that are far enough away from the others to question whether they originated from the same distribution or "set." We conclude Part 4 by addressing two very useful techniques, initially developed in industry, which allow us to formally assess the quality and safety of healthcare: **failure mode and effects analysis (FMEA)** and **statistical process control (SPC)**. FMEA is a structured method of **brainstorming,** using **subject matter experts (SMEs)** to identify IN ADVANCE all of the possible ways that something can go wrong (failure modes). **Statistical process control** is a graphic assessment tool that demonstrates an outcome measure evaluated over time (such as monthly wound infection rates or monthly readmissions after hospitalization for congestive heart failure). Using an initial pilot set of data, parameters are calculated for the process, allowing the determination of upper and lower control limits (typically three standard deviations above and below the mean or median value). A set of validated rules (**Western Electric rules**) allows major deviations in the metric to be identified immediately, triggering prompt assessment and correction.

Finally, we include a "focused" set of references. This text is NOT intended to be a comprehensive treatise on analytics, nor does it include a complete, up-to-date list of every conceivable reference. Rather, it is intended as a useful guide for physicians to understand and apply modern analytic techniques to the evaluation and improvement of healthcare delivery. So the references are intended to provide the next step of granularity, with the references in the references as the comprehensive compendium.

Additional materials—Many of the concepts and terms used in this book will be new. Accordingly, there is a glossary of terms. While it is not "comprehensive," it defines all of the terms that are highlighted in bold and hopefully most of the terms you will need to know. Additionally, a "Google search" of additional terms will provide definitions and material to review. When searching for material relating to "R," adding the term "CRAN" as a Google search term will focus the search. Minitab also has an extensive glossary of statistical terms, Help:Glossary.

This book contains both a bibliography and a set of references. The Bibliography lists textbooks which informed the development of much of this material and will be helpful in your general understanding. Many of them are available electronically through university libraries. The References section at the end of each chapter provides more detailed reference articles to selected topics. Extensive bibliographies are also available in the corresponding sections in the textbooks listed in the Bibliography. Most of the traditional reference materials for the analytics materials contained in this book are NOT available in medical libraries or medical references, so there has been no attempt to provide all articles or the "definitive article" on a particular subject. The goal has been to provide the next level of granularity to the interested reader.

R packages—A table of R-methods described in this book is included, together with the name of the appropriate package and the hypertext link to the R reference. With R opened, the command "library(help=package_name)" typed into the R-Console will also provide a summary of the methods included in the package. "help(methodname)" will provide a more detailed description of the method and its use.

1.3   Review of Introductory Concepts

1. Reliable and valid **METRICS** (formal, systemic, and standardized measurements) result in DATA—columns and rows of numbers in a spreadsheet, for example. In order for the data to be understood, some transformative process needs to be applied to convert the data to INFORMATION—a level of meaning to the data. In order for the INFORMATION to be usable, it must be incorporated into a context and thus becomes KNOWLEDGE. Further transformation of knowledge, by synthesis, interpretation, feedback, and learning, eventually results in WISDOM. Wisdom includes values, attitudes, and contextualization. This sequence of development from data to information to knowledge to wisdom, with a transformation process at each step, is often referred to as the DIKW model or hierarchy [10].
2. By now, we have all developed an uncanny ability to understand even subtle aspects of graphs and charts BY SIGHT. Not spending sufficient time graphing and visualizing data frequently leads to major errors in understanding or interpretation [11].
3. Recall that the scientific method starts with an idea, and that idea is immediately turned around into the negative of the idea—the **null hypothesis**. For example, suppose we believe that there is a **predictive relationship** between number of

complications and hospital length of stay which we then make a null by saying that there is NO DIFFERENCE. We then apply statistical methods to the data in an attempt to disprove the null hypothesis (which would be that THERE IS a difference). In order to do this, we have to decide up front how willing we are to be wrong. **And I have just redefined the meaning of p < 0.05.** No, it doesn't mean important, or useful, or even reasonable as is often believed. $P < 0.05$ simply means **I am willing to be wrong in rejecting the null hypothesis up to once in 20 times**. ("There are different kinds of probability … the extent to which an event is likely to happen and the strength of belief that an event is likely to happen. Although these are clearly rather different, the curious fact is that they can be represented by the same mathematics" [12]). As a comparative analogy, consider how often the weatherman is dead wrong in predicting tomorrow's weather and how we feel about that when we have worn the wrong clothes. Now that we have rejected the null hypothesis, and accepted the alternate hypothesis (that there IS a difference), it is critically important to realize that we didn't actually PROVE the alternate hypothesis nor did we even formally verify that the alternate hypothesis we chose is necessarily the appropriate alternate hypothesis. All we have "proven" (with a defined willingness to be wrong) is that we reject that there is NO DIFFERENCE, which means there likely IS a difference. But we will be wrong about once in 20. Putting that into a more quantitative perspective, the likelihood of flipping heads four times in a row is 1 in 16, which happens not infrequently. "Uncommon" events actually happen—and regularly [12]. Said in another way, based only on the accepted p-value concept, a journal with 20 articles per issue will have at least one random observation in two out of three issues. Which articles?

4. The Gaussian, bell-shaped distribution is called the normal distribution because, in the late 1800s and early 1900s, people actually thought that it described much of our world, thus "normal." However, it soon became apparent (although not to some!) that many things in the world DO NOT correspond to a symmetrical, bell-shaped curve. (Normal does not usually describe the real world, although it IS a setting on a washing machine!) Other distributions are more appropriate in these cases. One way to handle data that don't fit a "normal" distribution is to find a suitable mathematical relationship (known as a **transform**) to convert the data into a symmetrical pattern. Many software packages include routines for determining the needed transform to accomplish this.

5. A big issue that creates confusion is **cause and effect**. The only TRUE method of determining causation is a prospective, randomized controlled trial (PRCT). In such cases, all of the **covariates** can be controlled in the selection process and evened out by randomization so that only the variable of interest is being studied—either "it does" or "it doesn't." In spite of "wishing and hoping" to the contrary, there really isn't any way to DEFINITIVELY establish causation using retrospective data. Prospective evaluation is **deductive** and can lead to a conclusion, whereas retrospective assessment can only be **inductive** and so leads to an inference or a likelihood. Therefore possible causation in a retrospective data mining or analytics process must be assessed cautiously and tentatively. Since

particularly in quality and safety work randomization may not be ethical we must develop reliable ways to estimate whether causation is "reasonable," rather than accepting *p*-values alone. If a cause-and-effect relationship really isn't obvious, then it likely isn't true, even if it's statistically significant!

6. Often the goal of outlier analysis is to identify things that can be deleted (to improve the consistency of the data). It is critically important to understand, however, that outliers may actually be important and need to be evaluated further rather than deleted. Methods to identify outliers as well as to analyze them are both critically important.

7. Procedural rules and structure are critically important in brainstorming to assure that participants feel that the process is SAFE; otherwise they tend to withhold less popular ideas. The brainstorming process generates a list of potential failure modes and then uses a **modified Delphi process** to assess the likelihood, severity, and undetectability of each failure mode, to be used in prioritization.

8. Parametric statistics, those which underlie the typical medical publication, require that observations are "iid" (identical and independent distributions). This requirement is often not met, as distributions are regularly not identical and only rarely do medical observations have no correlation.

References

1. Jamshidi M. Systems of systems engineering: principles and applications. Boca Raton, FL: CRC Press; 2008.
2. Juran J. The upcoming century of quality. Qual Prog. 1994;27(8):29.
3. Masaaki I. Kaizen (Ky'zen), the key to Japan's competitive success, xxxiii. 1st ed. New York: Random House Business Division; 1986. 259 p.
4. Osayawe Ehigie B, McAndrew EB. Innovation, diffusion and adoption of total quality management (TQM). Manag Decis. 2005;43(6):925–40.
5. Reason J. Managing the management risk: new approaches to organisational safety. Reliability and Safety in Hazardous Work Systems. Hove: Lawrence Erlbaum Associates; 1993. p. 7–22.
6. Kaynak H. The relationship between total quality management practices and their effects on firm performance. J Oper Manag. 2003;21(4):405–35.
7. Crosson FJ. The accountable care organization: whatever its growing pains, the concept is too vitally important to fail. Health Aff. 2011;30(7):1250–5.
8. Cotter TS, editor. Engineering analytics-a proposed engineering management discipline. Proceedings of the international annual conference of the American Society for Engineering Management; 2014.
9. Porter ME, Lee TH. The strategy that will fix health care. Harv Bus Rev. 2013;91(12):24.
10. Ackoff RL. From data to wisdom. J Appl Syst Anal. 1989;16(1):3–9.
11. Tufte ER. The visual display of quantitative information. 2nd ed. Cheshire, CT: Graphics Press; 2001. 197 p.
12. Hand DJ. The improbability principle: why coincidences, miracles, and rare events happen every day, vol. xii. 1st ed. New York: Scientific American/Farrar, Straus and Giroux; 2014. 269 p.

Part I
Managing Data

Chapter 2
Data and Types of Data

Scenario
Juanita Sanchez is a PhD systems engineer, working as a data analyst for a large teaching hospital. She has been tasked with creating methods of visualizing large datasets to facilitate the decision making of the hospital board. In analyzing each of the variables in the large dataset, she notes that a number of the variables are not normally distributed and that many are highly correlated. She uses computer software to identify appropriate transforms to make the variables "normal" and she creates plotting methods to graphically demonstrate the individual variables and their interrelationships (**visualization, distribution identification, normalizing transforms, assumptions of statistical methods**).

2.1 What Are Data

Data are isolated facts, usually in a numeric format. Data are usually collected for a purpose. Since the introduction of computers into everyday life (in the mid-1960s, roughly) insurance companies, hospitals, and even medical offices have been amassing **databases** (structured collections of data). Within the past decade, people have been asking the important question "what am I going to do with all those data!" The implied real question is what can I do with the data to better understand what HAS happened and/or to predict what WILL happen. The field of analytics (actually a combination of applications including data mining, optimization, database management, applied statistics, predictive modeling, etc.) has evolved and matured and is considered synonymous with finding answers to these questions [1, 2]. The manipulation of raw data **transforms** the data into **information** by establishing context and relationships. Additional transformations applied to information, developing understanding and prediction capabilities, generates **knowledge**. Taking knowledge to a

© Springer International Publishing Switzerland 2016
P.J. Fabri, *Measurement and Analysis in Transforming Healthcare Delivery*,
DOI 10.1007/978-3-319-40812-5_2

Data- signs and symbols which have no
usefulness until augmented and transformed

Information- data augmented by "who, what,
when, where, why"

Knowledge- information which has been
processed, structured, organized or applied

Wisdom- knowledge augmented by judgment
and values

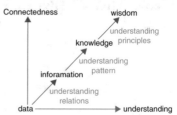

Fig. 2.1 The DIKW hierarchy represents the progressive development of conceptual learning, from data to information to knowledge to wisdom. Each step requires a formal transformation, typically as depicted here. It is important to recognize the stage of development of a concept in the DIKW hierarchy

higher level of awareness, interfacing with other knowledge sources, synthesizing new concepts, and developing new understanding are called **wisdom**. This progression, data-information-knowledge-wisdom, the DIKW hierarchy (Fig. 2.1), represents a widely held **epistemology** (how we know what we know) of the learning process [3]. Analytics focuses on the series of transformations that allow this hierarchy to develop and proceed, working through this sequence of steps using defined, often elegant, transformation methods. But the process requires spending a substantial amount of time (perhaps as much as 2/3 of the total time) on <u>understanding and visualizing</u> the data. It is tempting to proceed immediately with a set of data to the "fun" steps of computer modeling. But as the old saying goes, GIGO, garbage in-garbage out. Time spent in understanding, cleaning up, correcting, and visualizing data will result in better models, better understanding, and more useful predictions.

Data can be generated in two basic ways: prospectively, as in a designed experiment, where the investigator determines in advance what will be measured, what will be controlled, and what statistics will be applied, or concurrently/retrospectively, where the data are generated as a by-product of an activity, often collected in databases, and analyzed after-the-fact to allow understanding or prediction. Although the data can "look" similar, there are important differences in these two types of data – differences that are critical to the reliability and validity of the conclusions that are reached [4]. In the case of prospective data collection and analysis, the null and alternate hypotheses are established BEFORE the data are collected. They are "unique" to those data and they ARE the question. If the null hypothesis is rejected, there is only one alternate hypothesis. When using data from a database, the null and alternate hypotheses are determined AFTER the data are acquired and typically after an initial review of the data. They are chosen from an essentially unlimited number of potential hypotheses that could have been generated. If the null is rejected, the only confident conclusion is that the null is rejected. Thus the first step in approaching a set of data is to clearly establish which of these two approaches produced the data, as this has importance in establishing and interpreting the "hypothesis." If prospective, the hypothesis is clear and the alternative hypothesis defined. If retrospective, the hypothesis is actually one of many and the alternative can only be inferred.

2.2   How Are Data Structured

Data can be characterized in a number of ways [1]. Data structurally exist in four fundamental forms (Table 2.1), and understanding these is important to be able to know how each type of data can be used. Data can be names of things, **nominal** data. Since there is no numeric value to names, no actual computation can be performed. Nominal data can only be listed, sorted, described, and counted. Absolute frequencies, relative frequencies, percentages, and categories are all possible. Equations and mathematical models are not. It is tempting to try to do math, particularly when the original names have been replaced by numbers [1–4]. But these apparent numbers are NOT actual numbers, just new names that look like numbers. This becomes more of a concern when there is an order to the names, **ordinal** data. Ordinal data contain some element of size, smaller to bigger, slower to faster, lighter to heavier. Examples are the sizes of shirts: small, medium, large, and extra-large. These can even be replaced with numbers, sizes 6, 8, 10, 12, and 14. (Note, "french" sizes of catheters are actually measurements, while suture, needle, and scalpel sizes are not.) While it is tempting to use these apparent numbers in doing computations, they are still only names, just with a sense of order. This dilemma is frequently seen in evaluating survey-based data in which individuals select from "strongly disagree, disagree, neutral, agree, strongly agree" or some variation. When in word format, it is easy to see that the difference between strongly disagree and disagree is unlikely to be equal to the difference between disagree and neutral. But when the words are replaced by 1, 2, 3, 4, 5 it is easy to surmise that mathematics and statistics are possible. In fact, computers will not

Table 2.1 Classes of data

Nominal	Names of objects
Ordinal	Names of objects with implied size
Interval	Continuous data referenced to an arbitrary zero
Ratio	Continuous data referenced to an actual quantity

All data are NOT the same, meaning that the type of data defines what type of analysis is appropriate. Nominal data are simply names and can only be counted. Ordinal data have a sense of order but are still names, with much continuing controversy about what analyses are possible. Interval data can appropriately be analyzed by many approaches, but not all. Ratio data can be subjected to all mathematical manipulations alert you that these are not actual numbers. Ordinal data can be compared, <u>relative</u> magnitudes can be ascertained, and semiquantitative differences can be established. But not models. Nominal and ordinal data are qualitative and descriptive.

Quantitative data exist in two forms, and the difference is important. In the first form, **interval** data, there is a real numeric scale with exact differences between individual steps in the scale, but the scale does not correspond to a physical entity and does not have a true "zero" yet does have uniform intervals. As an example, temperature on either the Fahrenheit or Celsius scale is real and quantitative, but there is no actual <u>physical</u> meaning to 72 °F. It only represents a relative but quantitative difference between the freezing point and boiling point of water. The square root of today's outside temperature, while it can be calculated, is meaningless. Many examples exist in medicine, wherein a quantitative scale has been created based on a convenient yardstick that reflects "an interval relationship" rather than a physical entity: MCAT and USMLE scores, board scores, body adiposity index, etc. The second type of quantitative data, known as **ratio** data, are real numbers, and they are referenced to an actual zero value. This difference affects what types of mathematical manipulations are possible. ALL usual mathematical processes can be used with ratio data. So to put this into perspective, it is important to verify the characteristics of the data. There is almost nothing that can be done with nominal data except to count frequencies. Ordinal data can be compared to another grouping of the same data or, of course, can be counted. Interval data can be added and subtracted (since each datum represents a point on a somewhat arbitrary scale we can measure changes along that scale). Only ratio data are amenable to the full range of mathematical functions. It is important to realize that many medical data variables (for example scores, survey results) are NOT ratio data and can only be subjected to a limited number of analytical methods.

Another way to look at numerical data is in reference to a dimensional space within which the data "live." We are used to a three-dimensional space, referred to as Euclidean, which contains REAL numbers, both rational (whole numbers) and irrational (decimal points or fractions to the right of a whole number). There also exist imaginary numbers but we will not concern ourselves with these. Our senses are comfortable in 1-, 2-, and 3-dimensional space, but it requires a true "leap of faith" to deal in 15-dimensional space, for example.

2.3   Visualizing Data

The human eye has a remarkable ability to identify patterns and shapes. Often it is superior to a computer analysis (the computer might indicate that "something is there statistically," but it doesn't amount to much!). Using multiple approaches to visualizing the data will provide a detailed picture of what the data contain [5]. First, looking at the data themselves will identify missing values, outliers, and errors. Then, creating histograms, bar charts, and scatterplots will visually identify what the data "look like." Finally, descriptive statistics and correlation matrices followed by normality testing will "fine-tune" the understanding of ranges, collinearity, and normality, respectively. Methods for achieving these are discussed fully in the next chapter.

References

1. Tan PN, Steinbach M, Kumar V. Introduction to data mining. Boston: Pearson-Addison Wesley; 2006. p. 22–36.
2. Cios KJ, Pedrycz W, Swiniarski RW. Data mining methods for knowledge discovery. New York: Springer Science & Business Media; 2012. p. 2–7.
3. Ackoff RL. From data to wisdom. J Appl Syst Anal. 1989;16(1):3–9.
4. Matt V, Matthew H. The retrospective chart review: important methodological considerations. J Educ Eval Health Prof. 2013;10:12.
5. Tufte ER. The visual display of quantitative information. 2nd ed. Cheshire, CT: Graphics Press; 2001. 197 p.

Chapter 3
Software for Analytics

Scenario
Stephen Adams is a fourth-year medical student. As an undergraduate, he was a "computer whiz" and actually worked for a computer start-up company between college and medical school. He has been asked to work with a team to develop a course for last-semester seniors to prepare them to understand and apply data. They had an "evidence-based medicine" course in year 2, but the dean feels that understanding the modern medical literature requires a higher level of understanding—but not formal training in statistics. Stephen recommends using readily available software as the focus of the program: advanced Excel (spreadsheets, initial examination, descriptive statistics, add-ins); Minitab (menu-driven sophisticated statistics and modeling with excellent graphics); and R (powerful modern computer modeling and analysis, rapidly becoming the "industry standard.")

3.1 Initial Overview of Software

Modern analytics is highly dependent on readily available powerful computers and computer software. Although numerous packages of statistical software are available, only a few are required to do high-level analytical work. Though it may seem premature to address specific computer software already, understanding some of the capabilities of computer software from the beginning will facilitate learning analytics. I generally use three software packages for analytical modeling, a spreadsheet package, a menu-driven statistical package, and a "specialty" package, moving the data from one to the other as needed. While many examples exist of each, we will focus on Excel for spreadsheets, visualization, and initial statistics; Minitab for routine statistics (although other menu-driven statistical software will be analogous); and "R" for very advanced methods (although SAS will perform many of them).

© Springer International Publishing Switzerland 2016   19
P.J. Fabri, *Measurement and Analysis in Transforming Healthcare Delivery*,
DOI 10.1007/978-3-319-40812-5_3

You probably already have Excel, so just need to activate add-ins; Minitab has to be purchased, but there is "freeware" available named PSPP; R, RCommander, and RExcel are all freeware.

Modern computer software can greatly simplify the task of analyzing medical data. Software can be thought of as having a "back end" (where the actual calculations occur) and a "front end" (what is seen on the screen, the user-interface). The back end is pretty constant from software package to software package. Since visualization of data is so important in understanding and preparing, software that facilitates the initial visualization and data manipulation is helpful. Excel, already readily available in Microsoft Office, does that, and will serve as the "home" for the initial work on a data set.

3.1.1 Excel

Excel is known to just about everyone, as it is part of Microsoft Office, and has become the "de facto standard" in spreadsheets [1–5]. Opening an Excel file presents a "workbook," which contains a number of existing (and a much larger number of potential) worksheets. The individual worksheets are indicated along the bottom as tabs, whose names can be changed to improve understanding and organization by right clicking and choosing "rename." The spreadsheet typically consists of individual records (such as patients) in rows with individual attributes as variables in columns. This is the "standard," default format and will be used throughout this book—variables in vertical columns and records in the rows.

Although Excel, and other spreadsheet software, now makes it possible to make spreadsheets "pretty" (colors, merging, symbols, etc.), avoid adding additional formatting to the spreadsheet. When data are copied and pasted or exported/imported from a spreadsheet into another software package, these extraneous formats are often not recognized and completely stop the process. Spreadsheets work most efficiently when they have simple, lower case variable names in the top row, and continuous columns of data beneath them. Some secondary software packages are case sensitive, so only using lower case avoids having to remember if capitals were used in a word. Also avoid complex or lengthy names to avoid error because of the need to type them over and over. Never place anything in the space below the data, because if forgotten it will end up being included in computations. Simple is definitely better! Maybe not as "pretty," but much more functional.

One very important reason to always initiate analysis with a spreadsheet is that you can see all of the data. Data that have been stored within more advanced software packages are usually hidden and require "asking" to see things. I prefer to be able to see the whole data set in the beginning, and I can use many of the built-in functions of Excel to help me evaluate the data for error, duplication, etc. Long columns of data can be repositioned easily on the spreadsheet. I can also perform complex manipulations of the data as well as graphic visualization, all without having to leave Excel. Furthermore, there are now many advanced "add-ins" available that embed within Excel and greatly expand its capabilities. These can be found with a simple search, but I haven't found a need for anything other than what is covered here.

3.1.2   Menu-Driven Statistical Software

Different statistical software packages were designed with different users in mind, and the software is tailored to make life easy for these users. SAS, for example, is a very widely used statistical software package that was designed for the "hard sciences." SPSS was designed to be user friendly to social scientists. Minitab [6] was designed principally for engineers and the front end includes terms, applications, and formats that are commonly used within engineering. All of these, and many others, will serve admirably for doing straightforward statistical and analytical problem solving. Since Minitab was designed for applied and systems engineering, it is the most intuitive for the developing health systems engineer. However, if you prefer one of the other software packages, everything we discuss should also work with minor "adaptation." Help with the menu functions can be found by searching for the method plus the name of the software.

3.1.3   Advanced Analytical Software

"R" [2, 7–12] is a very modern and somewhat "eclectic" analytics software system. It was developed in the mid- to late 1990s by Ross Ihaka and Robert Gentleman and named "R" to reflect their common first initial. It is a statistical and visualization "environment" rather than a software package. In essence, and this is a gross oversimplification, R is a set of rigid computer standards and regulated "mirror" network servers, supervised by an international committee of experts who keep everybody honest. Home for "R" is known as CRAN (Comprehensive R Archive Network), which serves as a wonderful "Google term" to search for everything and anything. Anyone in the world can submit a proposed new package, as long as it follows the rules [10] and syntax. The package is submitted to the committee, compliance with standards is verified, and the package is thoroughly evaluated to establish that it does in fact work. Only then is it posted on the multiple, worldwide "mirror" servers and available FREE for download. The hardest part about "R" is that it's not "user friendly." Because the syntax and standards must fit a wide variety of areas, they are strict and rigid. There is no room for error. Over the past 15 years, extensive supplementary published materials have made it more understandable, but it's still quite difficult to use. The reason to use it is that it contains cutting-edge approaches and methods, enhanced weekly, that just can't be found in traditional "commercial" software.

3.1.4 Middleware to Make R Usable

An additional package, RExcel [13], was introduced in the last decade. RExcel serves as **middleware**, nestled between Excel and R. It provides menus, drop-down lists, and relatively easy data transfer, analysis, and visualization. In other words, it allows a very difficult system of packages to be much more intuitive and user friendly. Occasionally the link between Excel and RExcel becomes a bit unstable.

An alternative to RExcel is a package within R called RCommander (Rcmdr). Rcmdr is found within the list of R packages. An advantage of Rcmdr over RExcel is that RExcel only works with 32-bit Excel while Rcmdr will import an Excel file from 64-bit Excel, avoiding the need to obtain another version of Excel if you are using 64-bit Microsoft Office. Once R is downloaded from the CRAN website, the Rcmdr package can be installed directly from the GUI interface known as RConsole. Once loaded, the command library(Rcmdr) will automatically load a large number of sub-sidiary packages and files, and will open RCommander. If your Excel file was prop-erly prepared (data in columns, lower case variable names in the top row, no extraneous material) and saved on the desktop, clicking on Data:ImportData:fromExcelFile will open a pop-up that prompts naming the file within R. It is simplest to repeat the file name used to save the Excel file (use lower case and no symbols!). Select the appro-priate worksheet and it will be saved within the R environment. The commands in the top menu of RCommander will now work on the incorporated Excel spreadsheet. An additional advantage is that both RConsole and RCommander can be used concur-rently, although the results of a command will only appear in the window that was used to initiate it.

We will revisit these three software systems repeatedly, but to summarize, Excel is a wonderful place to store, evaluate, visualize, and conduct initial analysis and graphics. Data can then be "pushed" into other software environments for more advanced work. Whenever possible, pushing into commercial, menu-driven soft-ware, such as Minitab (or PSPP), is the easiest approach. In addition, Minitab pro-duces a large number of graphs and charts as part of what it routinely does, which greatly facilitates understanding and communicating. But when the commercial software won't do what really needs to be done, the data are pushed into R by using RExcel or Rcmdr, which allows "state-of-the-art" modeling and analysis. We will now look more closely at each of these platforms.

3.2 Excel (and Concepts Essential to Using Excel)

Excel "grew up" with the introduction of Excel 2007. It now will hold over 16,000 columns and over a million rows PER WORKSHEET. Only the largest datasets cannot fit. In addition, built-in "wizards" help to insert data into Excel in the proper format. Raw data files exist as either "delimited" (some character— often a comma or a space—separates the individual entries) or "fixed width" (all fields are a specified number of spaces wide). Data that are not already in Excel format are commonly packaged as comma-separated variable (CSV) files (the column separations are commas; the row separations are semicolons). Excel can input either fixed-width or character-separated formats to simplify transferring data into Excel, but there are also predefined "import" functions for many existing database packages.

3.2.1 Excel as "HOME"

It is helpful to have a place where it is comfortable to begin an analytics problem. Once placed in an Excel workbook, data can be easily analyzed, modified, transformed, graphed, and thoroughly understood, all within a convenient and user-friendly environment. Although other analytics software have the ability to perform many of these functions, Excel is straightforward, capable, and standardized. When the dataset is cleaned up, visualized, and understood, all or part of the dataset can be "pushed" into more advanced software to accomplish specific tasks. If only selected columns are needed, they can be rearranged on a new worksheet page using copy/ paste, so that only the variables needed are included.

Spreadsheet Rules. It is best to adhere to the convention of names of variables in the top row, with data in columns, no extraneous material, and no capitals or symbols—just words (nominal variables) and numbers (continuous variables) in standard decimal format with the desired number of decimals. While not covered here in detail, there are many "core" Excel spreadsheet functions with which you should be familiar. In particular, **Paste special**, **values only**, and **transpose** are useful in moving data from one place or worksheet to another in their existing form or by switching row and column orientation. After identifying a range of data and clicking on "copy," a right click will allow choosing **paste special**, and clicking on paste special will paste only numeric values (copying only the numbers and not the equations or formatting). The transpose function has the exact same effect as transposing a matrix in linear algebra—rows become columns and vice versa. Of the very large number of commands available in Excel, the most useful commands for analytics, located in the top row of menu labels, are found under **"Home," "Insert," "Data,"** and **"Add-ins"**—useful because they contain the functions for cleaning, understanding, and visualizing data (Fig. 3.1, Table 3.1).

3.2.2 Some Useful Cell Functions in Excel

A cell function is typed directly into a spreadsheet cell and it performs even very complex calculations and manipulations of data from around the spreadsheet. A large inventory of prepared cell functions can be found by clicking "f(x)" in the

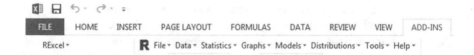

Fig. 3.1 The menu bar for the Excel add-ins "RExcel" and "RCommander." The menus allow menu-driven operation of "R" with a full range of analytical tools and graphic methods

Table 3.1 Toolbar menu bar in Excel

Menu	Drop-down list
Home[a]	Cut
	Paste
	Paste Special
	Conditional Formatting
	Find and Select
Insert[a]	Pivot Table
	Charts
	Equations
	Symbols
Page layout	
Formulas	
Data[a]	Sort
	Text-to-Columns
	Conditional Formatting
	Remove Duplicates
	Data Analysis
Review	
View	
Add-ins[a]	RExcel and others

[a]Useful for analytics

menu bar above the "C" column. Once learned, the functions can be typed directly into the cell, always beginning with "=," paying particular attention to appropriately "nesting" the parentheses which determine the order of calculation. Of particular interest, Excel includes a function, **=sumproduct**, which multiplies corresponding entries in two or more columns (or rows) and adds all of the products. It is analogous to a linear algebra function, the dot-product, except that dot-product multiplies a row vector by a column vector, while sumproduct multiplies two columns (or two rows). In both cases, the resultant is a scalar numeric representing the sum of products. This could also be used for the sum of squares, the sum of residuals, the sum of squared residuals, etc. In practice, this is a very useful spreadsheet function by avoiding having to create either multiply nested formulas or entering a long series of multiplied terms separated by pluses. The data ranges must be of the same length and the same orientation (row or column). With a little practice, this function will greatly simplify many spreadsheet tasks.

The function = sumproduct introduced the concept of vector multiplication. We have established the convention that data are always placed in columns, so each column can be thought of as a vector containing those data. However, each row represents an individual record, containing the appropriate element from all of the columns, so each row is also a vector. Correspondingly, a set of adjacent columns (vectors) represents a matrix, as does the same data thought of as rows. The concept introduced by "sumproduct" is at the core of vector/matrix mathematics—that is, performing a series of multiplications and then adding the results together. Modern software is able to perform vector/matrix operations much faster than if programmed to do the same operation stepwise, so matrix mathematics is very practical. It is analogous to the routine operations of addition, subtraction, and multiplication but with a few "rules": (1) adding or subtracting two vectors requires that they have the same exact dimensions and yields a result that also has the same dimensions; (2) multiplying two vectors or matrices requires a specific relationship between the number of rows and the number of columns and produces a unique result that depends on those dimensions; (3) division is not defined but can be accomplished functionally by multiplying with an "inverse"; (4) unlike regular multiplication, matrix multiplication is order specific, so we can matrix multiply "on the left" and matrix multiply "on the right" with different results. Matrices are defined by the number of rows and the number of columns (R by C or RxC—remember the mantra "row by column," as it governs everything that is done using a matrix). A vector can be thought of as a matrix with one of the dimensions being "1." The easiest way to remember the rule for matrix multiplication (RxC)*(RxC) is that the inside C and R must be the same, and the outside R and C determine the footprint of the result. For example, a matrix of 3 rows and 2 columns (3×2) multiplied by a matrix of 2 rows and 4 columns (2×4) IN THAT ORDER results in a 3×4 matrix. The 2s match and the 3 and 4 define the footprint. Note that if you tried to do it in THE OTHER ORDER (2×4) $\times$ (3×2), the inside numbers (4 and 3) don't match, so the matrix multiplication is not possible.

In Excel, matrix multiplication is an ARRAY FUNCTION, meaning that you must define the region (or footprint) IN ADVANCE by highlighting it and then type the multiplication formula (using the ranges of the two matrices IN ORDER) which appears in the upper left cell. As for all **array functions** in Excel, you must press Ctrl + Shift + Enter and the array will show the result. Note that to delete or modify any part of the array, you must highlight the original array, delete, and start over. It is not possible to modify inside a defined array. In fact, the array must be intact just to be able to delete it! Excel is not the easiest place to multiply matrices, but it is certainly available when you are working within Excel.

3.3   Menu Methods in Excel

This section focuses on a small subset of the many methods included in Excel
(Table 3.2). The methods and functions selected are particularly useful in the early
stages of data analysis and modeling. The selected methods will be addressed under
the menu tab where they are found.

3.3.1   HOME

Under the "**Home**" tab, you will want to be able to use "**Conditional Formatting**"
and "**Find and Select.**" Conditional formatting allows you to highlight in color
those elements in a massive spreadsheet that meet certain criteria. You can use

Table 3.2 Useful analytics
tools in Excel

Command	Drop-down list
RIGHT CLICK	• Cut
	• Copy
	• Paste
	• Paste Special
	• Insert
	• Delete
	• Sort
	• Format
Menu Item	*Sub-menu*
INSERT	• Pivot Table
	• Charts
	• Equation
	• Symbol
DATA	• Sort
	• Text-to-Columns
	• Remove Duplicates
	• Data Analysis (must activate)
	• Solver (must activate)
HOME	• Conditional Formatting
	• Find and Select
ADD-INS	• RExcel (must install)
	• RCommander (must install)

A click on the right mouse button will display the items on
the top row as a drop-down list
The four Excel menu items most useful in performing analytics are shown with the sub-menus

multiple colors or borders to allow looking at more than one criterion at a time. For example, you could highlight all negative numbers, numbers smaller than some minimum or larger than some maximum, etc. You can also highlight duplicate values or entries that contain text. While this may seem trivial when considering a very small dataset, when your spreadsheet contains 10,000 columns and one million rows, finding these abnormalities without visual clues is daunting.

The Conditional Formatting function highlights all of the cells that meet specific criteria, selected by the user. Clicking on Home:Conditional Formatting:Highlight Cell Rules displays numerous options for selection conditions: values greater than, less than, etc. Once chosen, all cells that meet the one or more criteria selected are highlighted in the selected color and border, allowing scrolling through the spreadsheet to identify where and how many. Find and Select is particularly helpful when you want to identify all of the cells that meet a specified criterion and replace them. For example, you might want to replace all negative entries with zero. Or you might want to change all zeroes to a very, very small decimal number to allow logarithms. Or replace a repeatedly incorrect entry. Within Find and Select, the Find function will step through them one at a time, unless you choose "all." Other useful Find and Select subfunctions include Replace—which can step through each appearance of a word or number or replace them all en masse—and Go To Special—which allows searching for specific types of items, such as Comments, Blanks, and Objects.

Both Conditional Formatting and Find and Select can be used to identify blank cells (missing values). We will discuss the rationale and strategies for dealing with missing values later, but first, we have to find out how many are there and where are they located. Conditional Formatting will highlight all of the blank cells, so that you can quickly estimate how many are there, where are they located, and the existence of a pattern. To do this, click on Conditional Formatting, then "New Rule," and then "Format only cells that contain." Click on the drop-down box labeled "Cell Value" and then click on "Blanks." At the lower right, click on the "Format" box and then "Fill." Pick a color, and then "Okay" twice. You will see all of the blank cells highlighted with your chosen color. Scroll through the spreadsheet looking for how many, where, and a pattern of missing values. This is a great way to find but not to fix. You might want to do this first to understand clearly the magnitude of the problem. As soon as you have completed this, use the back arrow to "undo" the conditional formatting before proceeding. "Find and Select" allows you to either step through the missing values one at a time or alternatively make a "repair" to all of them simultaneously. Click on "Find and Select," followed by "Go to Special" and then "Blanks." All of the blank cells will be highlighted in gray, with the cursor in the first blank cell. Enter a desired value into this cell, followed by "Enter" and you will step to the next blank cell. Continue serially until all blank cells have been addressed.

Most of the other functions contained in the "Home" menu are easily accomplished with a right mouse click (cut, copy, paste, paste special, insert, delete, sort, format). However, note that the "insert" reached with a right click allows entering a new column by displacing the other components of the spreadsheet in a specific direction.

3.3.2 INSERT

The **Insert** menu tab includes many useful tools (Pivot Table, Charts) not available with the right click. The right click "insert" and the Menu "INSERT" are complementary, not duplicative.

The **Pivot Table** function creates a "slice and dice" of the data. The term apparently originated with a very early database function that addressed the fact that databases don't allow you to easily look at the data without specifically asking for pieces to look at. The "slice and dice" function was created to allow honing in on the data variable by variable and row by column, as well as to do some simple tabulations such as counts, sums, averages, standard deviations, and more. After clicking on "Pivot Table," highlight a range of cells. For a moderate-sized spreadsheet, the easiest way is to click on the upper left cell, and then press the Shift key while clicking on the lower right cell (or vice versa). For very large spreadsheets, this can be accomplished either by clicking the lower right cell; then while holding the Shift key, scrolling up to the top with the right scroll bar and over to the left with the bottom scroll bar; and clicking on the top left cell. An alternative method, with a cell marked within your data range, is to just hold Control while pressing "A." The former allows you to clearly see what you are selecting, while the latter selects all of your filled-in spreadsheet.

After selecting the range of cells you wish to slice and dice, click on Okay and you will see a panel on the right side of the screen that allows you to control the slice and dice function. All of the column variable names will be displayed in a table. By clicking on the variables you wish to include for this run through the data, you will select the components that get sliced (analyzed as a function of one variable) and diced (analyzed as an intersection of two or more variables). At the bottom of the panel, there is a two-by-two grid (filters, columns, rows, values). The variables you selected will already appear under "values." At the right of each variable name is a down arrow. Clicking on it, followed by "field settings" and "custom," will show the many options available for the display (sum, counts, average, etc.) Select a value type for each variable, as appropriate for your analysis, or you can select "automatic" instead of "custom" and Excel will select a value type (which may NOT be what you want!). You can now drag and drop any of the variables from the value component into any of the other three zones. By dragging up to "columns," you select that variable for slicing. By then dragging a second variable to "rows," you create the dice. By dragging a variable to filters, you create a drop-down list at the upper left that allows you to create the equivalent of multiples of these two-by-two grids that you can move between. So it is possible to slice (select rows), dice (select rows, then columns), and/or segment into separate drop-down forms (select filters). The pivot table will display on a new sheet (helps avoid potential future errors) within the workbook unless you select "existing worksheet." Pivot tables take some practice getting used to, but once you are comfortable with them, they allow you to get a detailed understanding of the data. This is particularly useful in large datasets in which the "global view" is often insufficient.

Visualizing the data, as already stated, is a critical early step in handling a dataset. The **Chart** functions create a number of different types of charts and graphs to visualize selected aspects of the data. While each of them has a useful role in visualizing, most are intended for presentations. The scatterplot option is typically most valuable in developing a quantitative understanding of relationships and magnitudes. First select two columns by clicking the letter at the top of the leftmost selected column, and then with "control" pressed, the letter at the top of the rightward column. In the "charts" area, in the lower center, is a graph with multiple dots and a down arrow. Clicking on the down arrow produces a drop-down panel. The upper left scatterplot should be selected. If you selected the two variables of interest, you will see a new graph, which can be "spruced up" by clicking on various portions of the graph, followed by a right click. This allows adding additional names, ranges, or information. Note that the graph is on the spreadsheet that contains the original data. You can move it to the right, so that it is outside of the useful data range, or cut and paste it into a separate sheet within the workbook. Note that a new choice of options has appeared in the top menu area. These only change the appearance of the dots. However, if you move the cursor into the area of the data on your graph, right click and then click on Add Trendline; a panel appears on the right with a number of options. The upper portion allows you to do a mathematical transformation of the trendline equation from linear (default) to various other mathematical relationships, allowing you to explore other options. At the bottom of the panel are options for additional analysis, which change with different selections in the upper panel. Most useful is found when "linear" is selected, which allows the display of the mathematical regression equation as well as "R-squared." We will spend considerable time discussing R-squared, but for now, consider that it is the percentage of the total variance of the dots in the graph from the horizontal x-axis of the graph that is DUE TO the mathematical formula. For example, if R-squared is 0.14, that indicates that 14 % of the variance (in the y-direction) is DUE to the mathematical relationship and 86 % is noise. This may very well be enough of a relationship to be statistically significant, but it suggests that it is only a weak association and not a stronger, predictive relationship.

3.3.3   DATA

The **DATA** menu includes several functions that are useful in managing the variables in your spreadsheet: **Sort, Text-to-Columns, Remove Duplicates**, and **Data Analysis**. The Data Analysis tab is the workhouse of Analytics in Excel and will be addressed separately in the next section. We will begin with Sort, Text-to-Columns, and Remove Duplicates.

3.3.3.1   Sort

Selecting "**Sort**" allows a hierarchical, multilevel sorting of the datasheet based on selected variables in the top row of the spreadsheet. First, identify the columns or range of columns that you wish to sort. Typically, this will be the entire dataset, as sorting only part of the dataset will disorder your data. If you attempt to do this, Excel will warn you that there are adjacent data. Click on "SORT"—a pop-up screen appears. Make sure that "My data has headers" is clicked in the upper right and then click on the down arrow in "Sort By." This will display all of the variable names in the range you selected. Click on the first and most important variable in the sorting process. If you wish to then sort within that grouping by using a second variable, click on "Add Level" and repeat the process. You can continue to add levels in the sort, which may have been determined to be necessary during the Pivot Table analysis. The number of levels is limited only by the available memory in your computer. Typically, however, only two or three levels are necessary. To the right of "SortBy" you will see "SortOn" and "Order." "SortOn" allows the sort to be performed using numeric values or colors. "Order" chooses small to large or vice versa. Sort can be used in a number of useful ways: for example, after creating a new column of random numbers =RAND() gives a random number between 0 and 1 and this can be "dragged down" to populate the column with random numbers. Then use sort to create a random order to the original data. Selecting the first 50 rows, for example, produces a random sample sized 50. Sorting a binary column with values of 0 and 1 allows segmenting the dataset into two; sorting on last name followed by first name, age, or some other "finer" category allows a structured display of the dataset; and so forth.

3.3.3.2   Text-to-Columns

Often the original database will contain data in compound fields, such as data and time together and first and last name together. This combination of distinct elements makes data analysis difficult if not possible, so the combined element should be split into its components using **Text-To-Columns**. First, you will need to insert sufficient columns to allow the new variables to be split out. If there are two components (such as data and time), you will need to add one column to the right of the existing column (note that Excel will overwrite the leftmost column with the first segment of the split). Do this by clicking on the letter at the top of the right adjacent column, right clicking, and then inserting. A blank column will appear to the right of the column to be split. Click on the letter at the top of the column to be split and then "Text-to-Columns." A wizard will open which shows the selected data column. As previously discussed, select "delimited" and then next. Most often the delimiter will be a space, but it could be a comma, semicolon, decimal point, or other (such as an asterisk or an ampersand, in which case just type the delimiter in the box after clicking "other"). The next window provides an opportunity to adjust the format of each of the new columns. You may have an additional window, but most often click "Finish." The original column will have been split into its elements.

3.3.3.3 Remove Duplicates

Remove Duplicates is one of the easiest ways to find and remove duplicate values. A wizard will open and ask you to identify the columns of interest within a selected range of columns. Be careful before proceeding as the next step will find and delete all duplicates within the selected range. To develop an understanding of the number and significance of the duplicates, "Conditional Formatting" can be used (Highlight Cell Rules, Find Duplicates) and this allows stepwise decisions regarding delete or no delete.

3.3.3.4 Data Analysis

The workhorse of the **Data** menu is Data Analysis. This function may not be visible on your spreadsheet, but can be activated easily. Click on the File menu, then **Options**, and then **Add-ins**. The functions in the upper portion are currently active, the lower are present but not activated, and "browse" will identify additional add-ins that are already contained in Excel but inactive. Click on **Analysis Toolpack** followed by okay. In the upper right corner of the Excel "Data" ribbon, you will now see **Data Analysis** at the far right end of the menu ribbon at the top of Excel in the **Analysis** section. Click on Data Analysis and scroll through the contents, as most of the methods included are useful in data analysis.

Within **Data Analysis**, focus on the following methods: **Descriptive Statistics**, **Histogram**, **Correlation**, **Covariance**, **t-test**s (three methods), **ANOVA** (three methods), **and Regression**. Because they are so important for analytical work, they will be discussed separately in Sect. 3.4.

3.3.3.5 Solver

The concept of gradient optimization would require a separate book, but for inclusiveness a brief summary is included here. Gradient optimization is an advanced modification of a technique developed by Dantzig (simplex optimization) during and after World War II to optimize the transportation and availability of supplies and munitions. It was critically important in overcoming the Berlin Blockade after the war. Simplex optimization is founded on solving a complex linear algebra problem, made more difficult by including uncertainty (called slack variables). It was entirely based on stepwise row/column manipulation. Modern computers allowed a transition to a gradient ascent (or descent) method, essentially testing at each small increment which way is up (or down). As an oversimplification, imagine walking up a hill blindfolded, with a walking stick. Take a step and check which way is up. Repeat. As should be immediately apparent, if the hill morphs into two hills at the top, it is possible to reach the lesser of the two without realizing there is another, taller peak. So too with gradient optimization. But the speed of modern microprocessors allows millions of small steps, using one of a variety of complex search algorithms, so if initial examination of the **response surface** graph shows only one

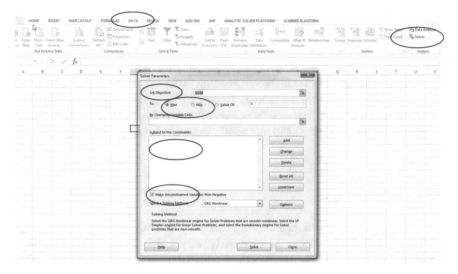

Fig. 3.2 The pop-up box for the Excel add-in "Solver" showing where the objective function, decision variables, and constraints are entered. The objective function is the mathematical expression of the eq. to be maximized or minimized; the decision variables are the unknowns to be "solved" to achieve the optimum; and the constraints determine the maximum or the minimum limits, traditionally based on resource availability. Clicking on "Solve" will run the optimization routine iteratively until it converges to an optimum

peak, Solver will find it. If more than one, repeating the whole process with different starting points usually identifies the global maximum. The structure of an optimization problem uses an "**objective function**" (the actual equation that is maximized or minimized, such as the equation for the sum of squared residuals) and a set of constraints (referred to as "subject to" or simply s.t.) that define the boundaries of the multidimensional area within which the search takes place. Solver is available in Excel, but must be activated through the Options menu (as described for the Analysis Toolbox). It is an extremely powerful and useful tool. The working screen for Solver can be seen in Fig. 3.2.

3.3.4 Add-Ins

Although the concept of Add-Ins was already introduced as Options that are already contained in Excel but need to be "installed," a separate menu tab called "Add-Ins" contains the link to "external" software that is added into Excel. It is typically identified by the suffix .xla in the file name. RExcel is an example of such an add-in. After installing RExcel, clicking on the Menu Tab "Add-In" will show at the left of the menu bar "RExcel." Clicking on it allows opening R and RCommander from within Excel by first clicking on "Start R," and then reclicking on RExcel followed by RCommander. For further details, see the Appendix.

3.3.5 Excel Summary

This section has introduced a number of Excel concepts and functions that are useful in analytics and are infrequently known. Excel can be an extremely useful tool for visualizing, manipulating, understanding, and performing initial analysis of large datasets. More sophisticated graphics, modeling, and statistical analysis are usually best performed in other software, with data being "pushed" from Excel. By routinely starting with data in a spreadsheet in Excel, many mistakes can be avoided, assumptions tested, and relationships identified PRIOR to developing complex analytical models. More detailed and in-depth explanations of Excel functions can be found in the sources in the Bibliography.

3.4 Returning to Data Analysis in Excel: The "Workhorse"

As discussed, Chart provides methods for initial visualization of the data. Data Analysis and Add-Ins that extend the capability of Data Analysis contain the Excel tools to perform analysis. Within Data Analysis (Table 3.3) is a set of 17 analysis tools.

Table 3.3 Excel data analysis tool pack

ANOVA: Single Factor
ANOVA: Two-Factor With Replication
ANOVA: Two-Factor Without Replication
Correlation
Covariance
Descriptive Statistics
Exponential Smoothing
F-Test Two-Sample for Variances
Fourier Analysis
Moving Average
Histogram
Random Number Generation
Rank and Percentile
Regression
Sampling
T-Test: Paired Two Sample for Means
T-Test: Two-Sample Equal Variances
T-Test: Two-Sample Unequal Variances
z-Test: Two Sample for Means

Once this add-in is activated in the "Options" menu in Excel, it will appear to the right of the menu bar in Excel. Clicking on it will open a pop-up menu showing the depicted commands

3.4.1   Descriptive Statistics

Descriptive Statistics is a single method that provides a wealth of information to aid in understanding your dataset. Click on **Descriptive Statistics**. Specify the range of cells either with Control and the letter at the top of each column or by clicking on the lower right corner of the dataset and dragging the cursor up to the top left. Next, click **Labels in First Row**, **New Worksheet**, and **Summary Statistics**. A new screen appears showing the results of a battery of statistical measures, but the columns are too narrow to show completely. Left click and hold on the leftmost column letter at the top, and then drag the cursor to the rightmost letter at the top, highlighting the area of interest again, but all the way to the bottom of the spreadsheet. Bring the cursor over to EXACTLY the vertical separating line between your leftmost and next columns, staying in the topmost row with the column letters. The cursor will change to a vertical bar and two arrows (which I will refer to as a cross-hair). Press the left click again and drag the cross-hair to the right until you create the column width that clearly shows all of the numbers. You will have increased the width of all of the columns you highlighted. If you wish, you can delete the columns that repeat the names of the methods to clean up the table. An alternative approach to widening a range of columns is to highlight all or some of the top (letter) row and double left click on one of the edge borders. The former method widens all of the cells to your chosen width. In the latter approach, each of the selected cells will be resized to accommodate its contents (variable sizes).

3.4.1.1   Central Tendency

The **Mean** is simply the mathematical average of all of the values in that column. It is a measure of **Central Tendency** (mean, median, and mode are all measures of central tendency). Keep in mind that your dataset represents a **Sample** taken from a "universe" of possible records, so it is important to think about how different other samples from the same universe would be. The central tendency can be thought of as the "middlemost" average value from a large number of potential averages, and 95 % of all of the averages should lie between plus and minus two **Standard Errors** (**SEM**). So the **Standard Error** is a measure of how much the mean might have varied on repetition, IF your data follow a "normal" bell-shaped curve. Excel does not have a cell command for SEM, but it can easily be calculated as STDEV(RANGE)/SQRT(COUNT(Range)). The **Median**, a distribution-free estimator of central tendency, is the middlemost element in the column—i.e., the same number of elements less and more. The magnitude of each element is unimportant, as this metric concerns itself with **Rank** in a series of elements. The **Median** is not affected by a tail in your distribution to the right or the left, as long as the ranks stay the same. The **Median** is thus insensitive to non-normality and is a better measure of central tendency in non-normal data. The **Interquartile Range** (IQR), which we will address later, is an estimate of how much the **Median** might vary with resampling, and is

conceptually analogous to the **Standard Error** of the mean. If your data are normally distributed, the **Mean, Median**, and **Mode** should all be the same. The Mode,
which is the MOST LIKELY value, is not very useful to us at the moment, except to
help affirm if the data are normally distributed. In small datasets, however, the
Mode may not be the same, so focus on how close the **Mean** and **Median** are.

3.4.1.2   Dispersion

The spread of the data can be assessed using standard deviation, interquartile range,
or range. The **Standard Deviation** (the square root of the **Variance**) is a measure of
the width of the distribution of the individual elements in that column. It is calculated from the sample you have, and is used in an attempt to generalize to the variability in the entire universe of all possible similar records. 95 % of all INDIVIDUAL
RECORDS should lie between plus and minus two **Standard Deviations** from the
Mean (in a normally distributed population). If your data are not normally distributed, the standard deviation still has some usefulness, but it <u>does not have the same
meaning</u>! Interquartile range can be used for non-normal data but must be calculated in Excel as this is not automatically provided. The IQR is simply the difference between the value at the 75th percentile (third quartile) and the 25th percentile
(first quartile). These quartile values can be determined using the = QUARTILE(range,
quartile) cell function, where quartile is an integer between 0 (minimum) and 4
(maximum), including the first, second (median), and third quartiles. Range is the
least "quantitative" estimate of dispersion, but it finds usefulness in some analytical
methods (for example, X-bar:Range process control). The **Range** is simply the difference between the **maximum** and the **minimum**. It is a very rough indicator of the
variability of a column of data, but the maximum and minimum themselves are
excellent indicators of high or low outliers, respectively, and are especially good at
signaling the presence of major data entry errors, as the maximum, minimum, or
both will be easily apparent as being out of the expected range for the variable.

3.4.1.3   Shape of the Data Distribution

When plotted on a frequency graph, data usually take the form of what is called a
distribution. If it corresponds to a mathematical function, it is known as a distribution function. Most available statistics are based on the presence of a symmetric,
orderly distribution, the Gaussian or normal. However, many data variables don't
actually fit that distribution. So defining whether a distribution is "normal" is a key
step in analysis. One way to assess normality is to look at the **Skewness** and
Kurtosis. Formally, the Mean is the "first moment" of the distribution, the standard
deviation the "second moment," skewness the "third moment," and kurtosis the
"fourth moment." Skewness should be thought of as a measure of asymmetry—does
the distribution have a long tail in one direction or the other. If there is no asymmetry, the skewness should be zero. Up to plus or minus 0.5 is acceptable. Between

plus or minus 0.5 and 1.0, there is moderate asymmetry, which SHOULD be addressed. Greater than plus or minus 1.0 indicates marked skewness and MUST be addressed. Asymmetry is usually managed with a suitable transformation of the data, often the logarithm, or by using statistical methods that are distribution free (nonparametric), addressed later.

Kurtosis is another way of assessing normality. Data that "fit" a normal distribution are not only symmetrical, but the height of the data distribution is "just right" for the width. There are two distinct methods to express kurtosis in statistical software and it is important to find out how a particular software package does it. To a purist, the expected value of kurtosis is 3. So in some software packages, 3 is the value to use (no kurtosis). But in many packages, 3 is already subtracted from the result. In Excel, then, 0 is the value to use. Between plus and minus 0.5 is okay. Greater than plus or minus 0.5 indicates moderate kurtosis (plus is called Leptokurtosis—too tall—and minus is called **Platykurtosis** or **Platybasia**—too flat). Greater than ±1.0 needs to be addressed.

Armed with this preliminary information, it should be possible to plan a systematic assessment of the data to find problems—outliers, erroneous data, or non-normality.

3.4.1.4   Correlation Matrix

Additional understanding can be obtained by creating a **correlation matrix**. First, however, let's introduce two terms which will be important throughout this journey: **input** (**independent**) and **outcome** (**dependent**) variables. While at first glance these terms seem self-explanatory, they are often misunderstood. Input and outcome, for example, may be perceived differently by the analyst than by the individuals who created the database perhaps decades ago. For example, estimated blood loss for a surgical procedure might have been included as an input variable as a consideration for looking at death or complications as outcomes. Alternatively, estimated blood loss could now be interpreted as an outcome variable as a consequence of medications administered. **Independent** is also used in two unrelated ways, so care is indicated. In a statistical sense, independent means that there is no relationship between two variables. In a data analysis sense, however, **independent** is used as a synonym for input or predictor, as opposed to **dependent** (outcome). In this latter sense, the word independent does NOT imply statistical independence from other variables. Armed with this understanding, we can begin our analysis of correlation by again looking at the full range of variables in the dataset, identifying for each variable its potential role as an input or outcome variable. In order to maintain the original relationships among the columns in the dataset, open a new copy of the data or copy and paste the data into a new worksheet in the current workbook. Move all of the columns that were indicated as outcome variables to the far right of the worksheet, using cut and paste. Delete the empty columns and also delete any columns that contain WORDS (you aren't changing the original dataset, so deleting is okay). All of the numeric variables identified as input are now on the left and as outcome on the right. Click on Data, then Data Analysis, and then Correlation in the drop-down menu. The pop-up window will ask for the data range. Enter all of the columns, both input and outcome. Verify that "Columns" and "Labels in First Row" are checked and click Okay. The correlation matrix will appear in a new worksheet. Split what you see into two separate "concepts": first the relationships among the input columns, and then the relationships between each input and the various outcomes.

A grouping of data into rows and columns is called an **Array**. An array can contain more than two dimensions (for example, a workbook with several worksheets, each with an identical number and type of rows and columns for different calendar years would be a three-dimensional array). A two-dimensional array that only includes numeric entries is specifically known as a **matrix**. Matrices have important mathematical properties, which we will address later. For now, consider that the Excel datasheet (with WORDS removed) is a matrix composed of the rows and columns. A correlation matrix in Excel is also a set of rows and columns, but with some empty cells in a triangular shape in the upper right. Note the identifying characteristics of the correlation matrix. First, it is square, which is to say that there is the same number of rows and columns. Second, the diagonal consists of only "1"s. Third, the matrix has triangular symmetry—the entries above and to the right of the diagonal of "1"s are the mirror image of the entries below and to the left (although in Excel and some other packages, the symmetry is indicated by leaving the upper right triangle of cells blank). Whenever you see a matrix that is square, has "1"s on the diagonal, and has triangular symmetry, it is a correlation matrix.

The correlation matrix is extremely useful in identifying and performing an initial assessment of relationships. The individual cell entries in the correlation matrix are the correlation coefficients between each pair of variables and range between −1 and +1 with +1 indicating perfect correlation, −1 perfect agreement in opposite directions, and 0 no relationship. The diagonal contains only "1"s because each variable has a perfect correlation with itself. Excel only includes the correlation coefficients for each pairing, whereas some software also includes p-values for each correlation coefficient indicating its statistical significance. For now, however, we are only interested in extreme relationships—those close to 0 (<0.1 indicating no relationship and probably independent) and those close to "1" (>0.9—strong relationship and collinear). Although the correlation matrix is often relegated to a "lesser" place in the statistical armamentarium, it is actually extremely important and useful at this phase of understanding and cleaning up the data and will help greatly in planning subsequent steps in analysis.

3.4.1.5   Covariance Matrix

Since we have addressed the correlation matrix, it is logical to next address the **covariance matrix**. It is also a square matrix (same number of rows and columns) and is triangularly symmetrical around the diagonal, but unlike the diagonal of 1s in the correlation matrix, this diagonal consists of positive real numbers which represent the individual calculated variances for each of the variables. The off-diagonal entries represent the individual covariance between each pair of variables and (unlike the correlation matrix, which is constrained so that values must lie between −1 and +1) the covariance matrix entries can be any value, very large or very small. The covariance matrix is not intuitive nor is it particularly informative, but it is an essential element of a number of mathematical transformations, in which case it is algebraically symbolized with a Σ (capital Greek sigma). Σ is more often used to indicate a summation, in which case it is located BEFORE the variables to be added, whereas Σ as the covariance matrix is most commonly located in the center of an algebraic formula. We will see the covariance matrix used in calculating Mahalanobis distance in matrix decomposition.

3.4.1.6   Histogram

The **histogram** function in Excel is cumbersome, but it's occasionally helpful to have the ability to do a histogram within Excel. The histogram function in Minitab and RExcel is much simpler as well as more useful. In Excel, it is first necessary to create a column of numbers to serve as the separation point between "bins." To create a histogram of probabilities, for example, which range from 0 to 1.0, I might type a 0 in the top cell, 0.1 in the cell below, highlight the two cells, and drag the lower right corner (known as the handle) down until the program generates 1.0. Now click on **Data Analysis**, followed by **Histogram**. The pop-up window will ask for the range of input cells. Specify all cells to be included, as was done previously, in the Input Range. Highlight the column of bin separators, just created. Clicking on Okay will generate the data for a traditional histogram. Clicking on Insert, the scatterplot icon in the upper menu bar, the down arrow, followed by the upper left scatterplot will display the histogram, which can be embellished by right clicking at various locations within the histogram. A different presentation of the histogram, known as a Pareto diagram, can be selected in the histogram pop-up menu. The Pareto format orders the bars in the histogram with the tallest to the left, decreasing in height to the right. The Pareto principle states that 80 % of just about any outcome is due to 20 % of the causes. In general, histograms are easier to perform in MiniTab or RExcel.

3.4.1.7   Methods for Performing Hypothesis Testing

Hypothesis testing is the underlying basis for all statistical inference. It can be performed with the assumption of a normal distribution using a parametric test, or using a nonparametric test which avoids the needs for the assumption. Excel provides only parametric tests: t-tests, ANOVA, and regression. A number of add-in packages broaden the statistical capabilities, and RExcel is a particularly useful statistical add-in. Within Data Analysis, there are three statistical functions that perform ANOVA, three for t-tests, and one for a z-test. What are these and how are they used? We will discuss hypothesis testing in more depth in a later chapter. In brief, hypothesis testing is intended to determine if there is a difference within a set of groups. We first identify the number of groups in the comparison and whether each group appears normally distributed using descriptive statistics. We initially "declare" a null hypothesis that both (or all) of the groups are really the same and whatever factor we are considering had no impact on the groups. Hypothesis testing is a method by which we then try to prove that our initial declaration (no effect) was <u>not</u> correct, with a predefined willingness (usually 5%, but it could actually be more or less) of <u>being wrong in rejecting the null (known as alpha—α)</u>. It is this likelihood of being wrong that is being assessed by these statistical tests—if the calculated likelihood of being wrong is smaller than our willingness to be wrong, we reject the null hypothesis and we reject our initial declaration of <u>no effect</u>, and we accept the alternative—that there IS a difference. Note that we don't actually prove that there IS a difference. We accept it as the alternative to NO difference, and we acknowledge that our decision to reject NO DIFFERENCE could be expected to be a bad decision 5% of the time.

Armed with a rough idea of what hypothesis testing is trying to do, and confident that a parametric test is appropriate because of known normality, we next define how many groups we're going to evaluate. If there are two groups, we will want to use a t-test. If there are more than two groups, we will want to use an analysis of variance (ANOVA). If there are x–y data pairs, some form of regression is probably indicated. Although they accomplish a similar task, t-tests, ANOVA, and regression come from very different mathematical families, with differing assumptions. T-tests are based on assessing means, ANOVA assesses dispersion, and regression applies ANOVA to a derived functional relationship. All three make a similar assumption that the data are normally distributed. Although the t-test starts with an assumption of a normal distribution of the data, if the two groups are similar in size and the standard error of the mean the t-test is "robust" to non-normality. (The standard error of the mean (SEM) is the standard deviation "adjusted" to address only mean by dividing by the square route of "n." SD applies to the dispersion of individuals; SEM applies ONLY to how much the mean might vary.)

3.4.1.7.1 The T-Test

The t-test compares the difference between two means using an estimate of dispersion (SEM). Since we don't know the TRUE mean and standard error of our samples, we estimate them from the data at hand, starting with the null declaration that there is NO DIFFERENCE allowing them to be lumped together to calculate a single standard error. The t-test then determines the distance between the means of the two groups (Δx) and divides it by the combined standard error of the mean (SEM), giving the number of standard errors that separate the two means. If the total sample size is greater than 30, a distance of more than two standard errors is unlikely (less than 5% chance) to have occurred randomly, so we reject the null hypothesis and declare that there IS a difference:

$$t = \Delta x \,/\, SEM$$

If the total sample size is less than 30, the necessary number of standard errors (value of t) will be larger than 2, up to 2.3. The exact number is based entirely on the total sample size and can be looked up in a table of t-values or in Excel for the desired rejection probability.

The three different forms of the t-test included in Data:Data Analysis accomplish exactly the same function but have slightly different assumptions. The **paired** t-test assumes that the two measurements were made in the same person, animal, test tube, etc. at two different times and we are looking at the difference WITHIN the same specimen. This is a stringent assumption and can't be violated. The **two sample** t-tests don't make this assumption—the groups are different but the same entity is being measured and compared. If the two groups have equal variability (the variance of one is less than two times the variance of the other) the **two-sample assuming equal variance** is appropriate. Alternatively, either because the ratio of the variances is greater than 2 or because we don't choose to make the assumption of equal variances, we can use **two-sample assuming unequal variance**. Even if the variances are actually equal, the result of both approaches should be similar, within the range of rounding errors. Unless you actually compare the variances, it is safer to choose unequal variance.

The **z-test** is analogous to the t-tests just described, except that the t-test was designed to address small sample sizes and the z-test presumes a very large sample size AND a known variance, from either scientific theory or prior measurement. Once the sample size exceeds 30, the t-test and the z-test in principle are the same. However, the z-test was designed to address a comparison with a known population mean and standard deviation rather than to compare two samples. Consequently, it is safer to stick with t-tests for comparing two sample populations and restrict using the z-test to situations in which a reference population mean and standard deviation are known and will serve as the basis of comparison.

Before leaving t-tests, it is important to reiterate that the t-test is based on measuring the difference between two means and comparing that difference to a standard measure of variability (SEM). Because it uses means, it is "protected" by a principle known as the central limit theorem, which makes it relatively robust to being used with non-normal data. This is quite different from the topic covered next, ANOVA, which does NOT use the mean, and thus is NOT protected by the central limit theorem from non-normality.

3.4.1.7.2 ANOVA

The ANOVA was a major contribution in the early world of statistics, introduced by Sir Ronald Fisher considered by many to be the father of modern statistics. Its purpose is to make comparisons which involve MORE THAN TWO GROUPS as well as comparisons in MORE THAN ONE DIRECTION. An often suggested alternative to the ANOVA is to perform multiple t-tests, assessing each and every possible pair. The problem with this is that the estimated likelihood of being wrong (alpha) will be VERY incorrect and apparent differences will be identified that don't actually exist.

A method to adjust this error is known as the Bonferroni modification. Although there are occasions when this approach may be appropriate and even preferable, for example with non-normal data for which the ANOVA may be ill suited, there are usually better ways to deal with >2 groups with non-normality. Thus, *t*-tests should be restricted to comparing two groups and ANOVA for more than two groups.

ANOVA literally means an analysis of differences in variance which essentially says it all. It does not compare means. It analyzes "widths." Consequently, to be accurate the data should be normal for the variances to truly represent the "width" of the data distributions. We will later address methods to "adjust" for non-normality, but first we will address the use of ANOVA using normally distributed data. Let's begin by referring back to the concept of the null hypothesis. If there is NO DIFFERENCE between the groups being considered, then they would all have the same variance since they came from the same population. So if the variability of the variances is within the range that would be expected due to sampling error, we accept the null hypothesis of NO DIFFERENCE. On the other hand, if the variability of the variances is greater than would be expected, we reject the null and accept the alternative—that there IS a difference somewhere. The actual test that underlies the ANOVA is known as the "F-test," which is simply the ratio of two variances (which we implied previously when discussing equal and unequal variances). Recall that a variance is typically estimated from a sample that is theoretically taken from a very large population. That sampling is subject to a concept known as **degrees of freedom (df)**. Interpreting the *F*-tests in ANOVA requires knowing the number of df overall and within each group. A *t*-test is "calibrated" using $n-1$ degrees of freedom. This is most simply described by saying that if I know that I'm going to sample "n" items, and I already "know" the average of the n items, then once I have sampled $n-1$ items, the last one is "known." While there are a few exceptions, it is generally safe to assume that df will be $n-1$. If a variable in a dataset has, for example, 100 entries and the average is "known," after considering 99 entries, the 100th is "fixed" by the average. So in a ratio of two variances, both the numerator and the denominator variables have a specific number of degrees of freedom, and the number of degrees of freedom for the two variances is important in assessing the meaning of the result of the *F*-test. Software will typically determine the df for you, but using tables requires knowing the number of df for the numerator and the denominator.

   Within Excel, there are three forms of ANOVA available within Data Analysis: **ANOVA Single Factor, ANOVA Two-Factor With Replication, ANOVA Two-Factor Without Replication**. ANOVA Single Factor (also known as one-way ANOVA) is analogous to a *t*-test with more than two groups EXCEPT that it is based on assessing variances and not means. It is "simple ANOVA." ANOVA Two-Factor is the simplest form of what might be called "complex ANOVA." (There are many forms of ANOVA, much more complex than Two-Factor, such as more than two factors, subfactors, hierarchical, and split plot.) Visualize a table with rows and columns. Along the top, the columns represent different levels of one factor (such as treatment regimens) and the rows represent **a second factor** (such as gender). ANOVA Two-Factor allows assessment of differences between treatments, differences between genders, and also the interaction effect of gender and treatment (is the treatment outcome also influenced by a difference in gender, yes or no). Each of these is, of course, subject to the assumption that the data are either normally distributed or can be mathematically transformed so as to be normally distributed. Although it is often said that the ANOVA is robust to non-normality, there **will** definitely be an error if the data are not normal, and the magnitude of that error is not known.

ANOVA: Single Factor can be visualized as a data table with more than two columns (representing groups) and multiple sample rows (representing individuals). Each group is SEPARATE AND DISTINCT from the others, representing discrete samples and not **repeated measures** in the same individuals. To begin, although Excel will allow you to proceed without this, it is a good idea to look at the Descriptive Statistics and affirm that the data in the groups appear normally distributed. When in doubt, there are formal tests of normality that will be discussed later (which also allow determination of which mathematical transform best "normalizes" the data). If the data appear normally distributed, proceed with the ANOVA by clicking on ANOVA:Single Factor. The pop-up window asks for the range of data, which represents the specific groups (in columns) and the individuals in each group (in the rows). Verify that "columns" and "labels" are checked, as appropriate. Alpha of 0.05 is the common default for how willing you are to be wrong, but you could enter a larger or smaller number. Clicking Okay will produce a table that appears in a new worksheet. At the top will be a "Summary," showing the names of the groups as rows and Count, Sum, Average, and Variance as columns. Count will verify the numbers within each group. Sum is not particularly useful, but even though the mean is not a component of the ANOVA interpretation, looking at the averages will give you a visual assessment of the comparison of the groups. As previously explained, the F-test (variance-ratio test) is the underlying basis of ANOVA. The variances in the last column are the variances of the individual groups, allowing an assessment of the degree of similarity of the variances among the groups. At the bottom is the ANOVA table. The rows show a **partitioning** of the **total variance** into calculated components that represent variability **between** the **groups** and variability **within** all of the **groups**. This is accomplished by measuring the **residuals** in several different ways. The residual is the difference between the value of a variable and its expected value, and the expected value is most often given by the average of the group of data. So a residual is typically the difference between an entry and the average for the specific subset of data. Squaring the residuals and summing them give the **sum of squared residuals**, also known as the **sum of squares** (SS). Dividing a sum of squares by the number of degrees of freedom (in this case, $n-$) gives a result known as **variance**, also known as the mean squared error (MSE). We will be exposed to many different forms of variances, but each variance is the sum of squared residuals divided by the appropriate number of degrees of freedom. We can thus calculate the sum of squares between groups as well as for within groups. The total-SS and the between-SS are calculated from the data, and the within-SS is the difference between them. Within-SS can be considered as the "error term." The first column ("SS") shows these sums, which when divided by degrees of freedom gives the corresponding variance terms or MSE. The next two columns display the df (the df for "between" is $k-1$, where k is the number of groups, and for "within" is $(n-k)$). The MS is the MSE for that subset. The F-test is the ratio of the two MS (MSE or variances) to assess significance, and the next column displays the value of this F (the MS-between divided by the MS-within). Adjacent is the calculated p-value for that F, given the two df, and the F-crit (critical value of F for the specified dfs) above which one assumes that there IS a difference somewhere.

Correct Determination of Sample Size in ANOVA. We have mentioned sample size, "n," and its corollary, degrees of freedom, "df." These must be known to conduct hypothesis testing. But sample size can easily be determined incorrectly unless we understand the difference between **Replication** and **Pseudo-Replication**. If I take a blood sample and measure the glucose level and then immediately take a second sample and do the same, I have two replicates, and I can consider the two results as being replicates. If, on the other hand, I take one blood sample but ask the laboratory to run it twice, I will get two answers, but I actually only have two measurements of ONE SAMPLE. In the former case, I am justified in saying that I have two replicates, but in the latter, I only have a single measure (which perhaps I know more "accurately" by taking the average). Erroneously counting pseudo-replicates can lead to a gross underestimation of how likely one is to be wrong (significance testing) because of magnification of the stated df. So the difference between the next two forms of ANOVA, with replication and without replication, is based on this distinction. Again imagine a table, this time with cells representing three columns (types of insulin) and two rows (once-daily and twice-daily injections). If many patients each had a single blood glucose, measured a single time, ANOVA with replication would be appropriate, with each cell containing a number of individual blood glucose measurements. On the other hand, if a single patient had each of the six combinations (types and times of dosing), but the glucose for each patient was repeated by the lab six times, there is only one measurement per cell, consisting of the average value of six measurements, and the ANOVA without replication is appropriate. For ANOVA with replication, the report is identical to ANOVA: Single Factor, except that there is double the number of tables—the ANOVA table includes rows, columns, and error, but with exactly the same determination. ANOVA without replication, which consists of only one value per cell, has a result table with row, column, and error, but the df represents only the number of rows minus one and the number of columns minus one. Since the total df is much smaller than the number of df in "with replication," the error term is divided by a smaller number of df. Pseudoreplicates exaggerate the number of df.

3.4.1.7.3 Regression in Excel

Regression is commonly used in the medical literature and is usually called "multiple regression" or less correctly "multivariate regression." There are three different ways to derive regression information using Excel, including one in Data:Data Analysis. Because the three methods are more closely related to each other than to other Excel functions, all three will be discussed here.

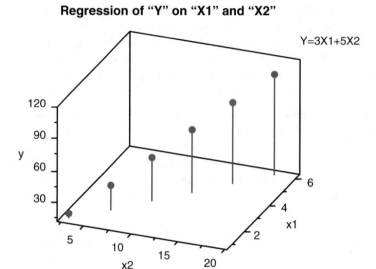

Fig. 3.3 A 3-D graphic depiction of the concept of "regression," showing individual points in 3-D space and the line that is the "best fit" to minimize the sum of squared residuals (errors)

Overview of Regression: Regression is a mathematical method which seeks to identify relationships between one or more input variables and an output variable. The term **"projection"** (Fig. 3.3) is often used because it essentially takes "a stick" which is directed into **"multidimensional space"** and looks at the shadow of the stick on one of the spatial axes. Regression is the relationship of the points on the line to their projection on an axis. A simple way to understand "projection" is to look at a blank wall while holding up a ruler. With the ruler fully exposed, the projection (relative to the wall) is the unaltered ruler. As the ruler is rotated, the appearance (and also the projection) changes, until, with the ruler "on end," there is nothing there but the end of the ruler. This relationship between the projection (one or more) and the corresponding value on a "vertical" axis known as "y" can be expressed as a mathematical equation consisting of an intercept and one or more slopes (coefficients) (Fig. 3.3).

Excel provides three different ways to derive regression-related data, but each serves a specific role: an enhanced graphic form within scatterplot (Charts) which provides a little detail about the best line; a cell function within the spreadsheet (=linest) which allows regression output to be used in other cell commands and calculations; and a separate window called Regression (Data Analysis) which provides robust and comprehensive multiple regression and ANOVA for analysis.

1. Scatterplot: The Scatterplot version can be obtained in three different ways after having created a scatterplot (Insert:Charts). Add chart elements by clicking on the +icon, followed by "Trendline," or by clicking Design:AddChartElements:T rendline, or by clicking Design:Quick Layout and selecting the small graph that displays f(x). Each approach will place the best-fit straight line in the chart, the

linear regression equation, and the value for R-squared, and is a quick way to identify a regression but it is limited to two dimensions. R-squared (the square of the correlation coefficient, r) is one of the simplest but also most widely applicable measures of "how good." For example, if "r" is 0.4, then R-squared is 0.16 and 16% of the total variability of the data can be explained by the model. Of perhaps more importance, however, is that 84% of the variability CAN'T be explained by the model. While formal interpretation is a bit more complex than that, particularly when there are many input variables, $(1-R^2)$ can be thought of as identifying the limitations of a model. We will later look at other, more complex methods of evaluating models.

2. =LinEst: The second method of deriving a regression model uses the cell command "=linest," followed by inputs. The syntax (string of entries) required is ("y" column, range of "x," yes/no for determining the intercept, and yes/no for complete statistics). This function is a "working" function that returns a range of answers (Array) in a specified format, so that each of the results can be used in subsequent spreadsheet calculations, in other words "behind the scenes." "=linest" is an **Array Function** which has some important peculiarities: Before entering the cell function, you must highlight a range of cells (the "footprint") large enough to contain all of the results; only numeric entries and not variable names should be selected; without touching any other keys, enter the "=linest()" syntax; press and hold the three keys Ctrl, shift, and then enter. An array of numbers will be displayed in the selected area, underlined. Details explaining this function and the key to understanding the array can be obtained through the built-in help function for "=linest."

3. Regression in Data Analysis: The regression method most useful in analytics is (Data:DataAnalysis:Regression). This requires that the selected variables be located in adjacent columns with "y" on the left and the "x"s immediately to the right. The resulting pop-up window can create very complex regression models if suitable transforms of each column of data are constructed within the spreadsheet (this is usually accomplished by creating for each a modified column using spreadsheet functions (square, log, etc.)). Then use Copy:PasteSpecial:Values to place the newly transformed variables into adjacent columns in a new worksheet. With Data:DataAnalysis:Regression selected, enter y-Range, x-Range, and check labels. Then click on the four options in "Residuals," followed by Okay. A complete regression analysis with ANOVA will appear in the new worksheet together with a large number of pop-up graphs. The report shows a lot of information. Multiple-R is a multivariate determination of the "overall" correlation. R-squared is the unmodified percent explained, while adjusted R-squared adjusts by the number of x-variables used and is more reliable. Standard error is the confidence interval (range of expected variability) for the predicted y (known as y-hat ($\hat{y}$)). The next section, ANOVA, shows the total sum of squared residuals being partitioned into components "explained" (regression) and "residual" (explained subtracted from "total"). The next panel provides statistics for each of the determined parameters: the y-intercept and each of the estimated coefficients. Assuming sufficient sample size, a value of "t" greater than 2 should be significant, as evidence

by the "*p*-value" and the displayed confidence ranges. The final panel lists the predicted values for each of the data points, the residual (observed minus predicted), standardized residuals in units of "z" (value minus mean divided by standard deviation), and the data to populate the cumulative probability plot. Of more value and interest, however, are the "residual" reports, including the plots that accompany the report (if selected)—a list of the residuals ($y - \hat{y}$), the same residuals standardized, and two sets of plots for residuals and line fit. Since the plots can only be two-dimensional, there will be pairs of plots for each variable (univariate), one showing the best-fit line and another showing the residuals. If the assumptions of linear regression are met, the residual plot should show an even distribution of dots going across. If the assumptions were not met, the residual plot will be wider in the center, wider on the ends, or some other deviation from "uniform across." Sometimes the axes selected by Excel result in a "crowded plot," which can be improved by changing the range of the axes.

3.5 Minitab

As described earlier, Minitab is the ideal third software package for health systems engineering as it was designed for systems engineers. It is fully menu driven and much more intuitive than R or Rcommander (Fig. 3.4a, b), plus it has some of the best graphics and visualization capabilities available. Each of the functions addressed here has excellent examples in Minitab by clicking "Help:Examples." In the top row of the Minitab display (Fig. 3.4c), the menu tabs show the various sets of options. If you use Excel for data manipulation and initial visualization, you will only occasionally use the "Data" and "Calc" menus since these functions are easily accomplished in Excel. However, you will find use for Data:Stack when you have several columns of like measurements (take individual columns and stack them in a single column, creating an index column from the column names) and Data:Unstack (take a long column and unstack it into separate columns using a column of categorical values as the index to accomplish the rearrangement). You will routinely use "Stat" and "Graph."

Under "Stat:BasicStatistics" (Fig. 3.5) most of the methods have already been described. "Normality Test" is a very useful function for determining if a column of data is normally distributed. There are three methods (Kolmogorov-Smirnov, the gold-standard; Anderson-Darling; Ryan-Joiner variation of the Shapiro-Wilks) which can generally be used interchangeably and work well for samples greater than 30. "Goodness of fit test for Poisson" is particularly useful for <u>small samples</u> where the measurement is counts.

"Stat:Regression" (Fig. 3.6) includes a full range of regression-based methods as well as logistic regression. Regression methods are used when the outcome variable in a model is a continuous variable and will be discussed under "Regression." Logistic regression is one of a set of classification methods, where the outcome variable is categorical: binary (two choices, e.g., 0,1), ordinal (more than two choices

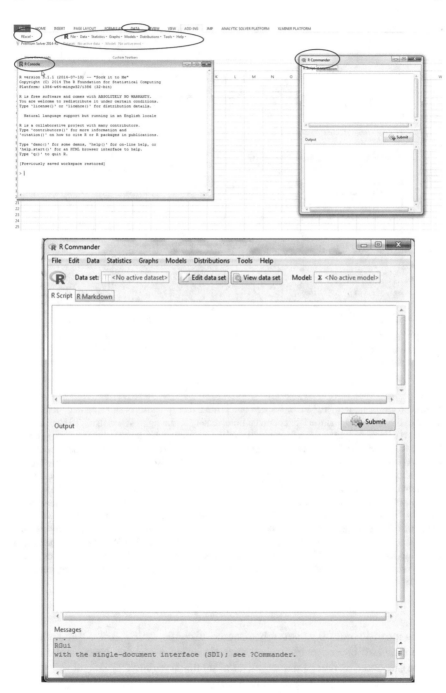

Fig. 3.4 (**a**) The Individual Consoles being displayed for RExcel and for RCommander. Opening "R" directly from the computer desktop will display the "RConsole" menu (on the *left*), which requires writing R-code for analytics, but it is particularly useful for installing and loading packages

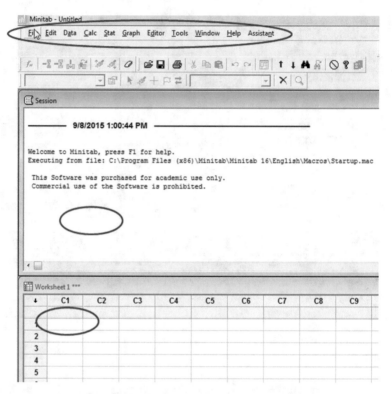

Fig. 3.4 (continued) into "R." In the background is the Excel spreadsheet showing that "RExcel" is active in the upper left and the RExcel menu immediately to the right. When using RExcel menus, results will be displayed in the lower window of the RCommander console (on the *right*) and the "transcribed" commands will show in the upper window. Understanding the transcribed commands is a good way to learn the R-code. Copying and modifying the displayed R-code can be used to run more advanced R methods that require key entry either into RConsole or RCommander. (**b**) RCommander can be opened directly from RConsole. It is initially installed using "Install Package" in RConsole. Once installed, typing library(Rcmdr) into RConsole will open the screen shown here. Note that the same menu shown with RExcel with the Excel menu bar is now shown at the top of RCommander, with the same two windows below. (**c**) The menu in Minitab is very similar to the RCommander menu. There is no need to type code, as everything in Minitab can be activated using the menus and drop-downs. The data spreadsheet is displayed below and can be imported or pasted from Excel. The results of Minitab procedure are displayed in the window between the menu bar and the spreadsheet

with an intrinsic order, e.g., strongly disagree, disagree, or 1, 2, 3, 4, 5), and nominal (more than two choices without any intrinsic order, e.g., blue, green, red). These will be discussed as part of the larger set of methods under "Classification."

"Stat:ANOVA" (Fig. 3.7) contains a full set of methods using ANOVA, including applications to linear models. However, most of the ANOVA output needed to evaluate a model is automatically provided in the results of a regression or classification method.

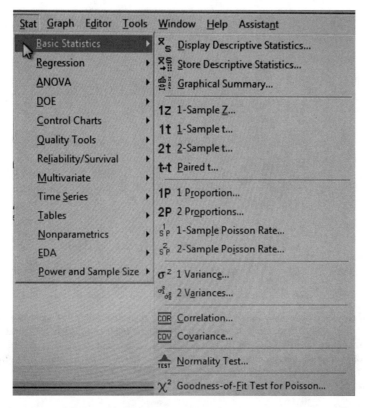

Fig. 3.5 Minitab Basic Statistics. By clicking on "Stat," the menu bar on the left is displayed. Placing the cursor (hovering) over "Basic Statistics" will display the menu on the right, showing all of the options for performing basic statistical evaluation

"Stat:DOE" indicates design of experiments, a specific engineering approach to highly structured analysis. While this is beyond our scope of interest, it is worth knowing that these methods can be easily found and applied.

"Stat:ControlCharts" focuses on different types of statistical process control models which will be addressed in Part 4. Statistical process control (SPC) is a combination of statistics and visualization that was first introduced as a set of tools that could be used in a manufacturing environment by individuals without advanced mathematics training.

"Stat:QualityTools" (Fig. 3.8) includes a large "toolbox" of methods used in industry which may find occasional use in healthcare. "Individual Distribution Identification" is very useful for exploring the possible underlying distribution of a column of data. This method provides standardized graphs and simple statistics, fitting the data to as many as 16 different distributions. If the plotted dots extend outside of the range contours and/or the p-value is <0.05, that distribution is not appropriate for the data. A "good fit" will have all of the plotted dots within the

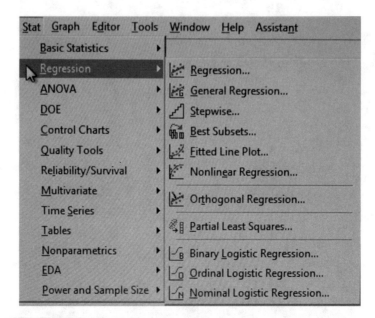

Fig. 3.6 Hovering over "Regression" in the Stat menu shows the full list of regression options. The *upper area* shows "traditional" regression options, including the ability to use "link functions" and to perform menu-driven nonlinear regression. Partial least square regression is a sophisticated method of "shrinking" the input variables. The *bottom area* shows three options for performing logistic regression, which is actually a classification method

range contour and a p-value >0.05. The Box-Cox option suggests a suitable transform to normalize the data.

In addition to reliability tests used in manufacturing, Stat:Reliability:Survival is useful for conducting survival-based analyses. Although the names of the methods are different from those typically used in medical survival studies, the actual methods are the same. Kaplan-Meier and log-rank are hidden here and will be discussed in Part 4, together with Cox proportional hazards, which is not supported in Minitab, although other types of regression-based comparative survival analyses are.

"Stat:Multivariate" (Fig. 3.9) includes a number of methods of importance in analytics: principal components analysis (PCA), factor analysis (EFA), cluster analysis (three types), and discriminant analysis. We will discuss cluster analysis and discriminant analysis later and will focus now on PCA and EFA. To create a context, remember that the dataset has variables in columns and records (or patients) as rows. The columns represent "variable space" and the rows "subject space." If we standardize our dataset (subtract the column mean from each element and divide by the column standard deviation creating a new "z-score" with mean $=0$, SD$=1$) and determine a covariance matrix, we have distributed the total variance as a function of the rows and columns but standardized on the columns. Even having done this, there is no assurance that the variables (columns) are independent of each

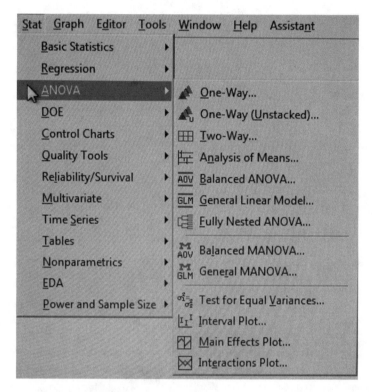

Fig. 3.7 Hovering over ANOVA displays all of the options for performing analysis of variance in Minitab. This is a surprisingly comprehensive array of options and should allow performance of ANOVA in just about any analytics situation

other (non-collinear). If we perform what is known as an eigen decomposition of this standardized covariance matrix (eigen refers to a set of essential and perpendicular vectors), we obtain a new set of variables (principle components) which are all perpendicular (orthogonal) to each other, meaning that there is NO correlation and they are actually independent. More importantly, the total variance that was partitioned in the covariance matrix is "loaded" onto these new variables such that the largest proportion is on PC1, then PC2, etc., with all variables being mathematically independent. The number of PCs is equal to the original number of variables. However, each PC has an associated number assigned to it (eigen-value) indicating how much of the original variance was loaded on that PC. PCs with eigen-values less than 1 make almost no contribution, so only PCs with eigen-values >1 should be retained. This results in a smaller number of new variables which are truly independent. The only problem is figuring out what the new variables mean. This is accomplished by looking at which of the original variables load onto each PC and assigning new names to them that represent what has loaded. What does this all mean? PCA is primarily useful for improving the mathematical analysis by creat-

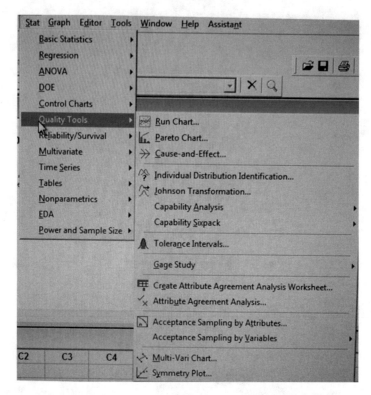

Fig. 3.8 Hovering over Quality Tools displays the menu on the right. Many of the options are useful in statistical process control. A particular interest in analytics is "Individual Distribution Identification" which will perform 14 different parametric distribution analyses plus 2 transformations (Box-Cox and Johnson). The Box-Cox transformation suggests the optimum transform based on the value of the logarithm. The Johnson transformation is a "jack-of-all-trades" transformation and will "fit" just about any set of data, but assigning and interpreting "meaning" are not possible

ing new variables in "variable space." To identify hidden or latent meaning, factor analysis is preferable.

To identify underlying meaning, factor analysis performs a similar process but in "subject space," largely overlooking the variance that is "common" or "shared" among all and focusing on the variance that is "special." This "special" variance is new groupings that contain "something in common," with the intent of providing some understanding of the "latent" factors within the data, this time from the perspective of "subject space." Often PCA and EFA will provide identical results. Some software defaults to using PCA for an EFA. What does this mean? If my goal is to clean up the mathematics, create truly independent variables, and reduce dimensionality, PCA will accomplish this. If my goal is rather to provide a level of deeper understanding of hidden factors underlying my dataset, EFA is the appropriate approach.

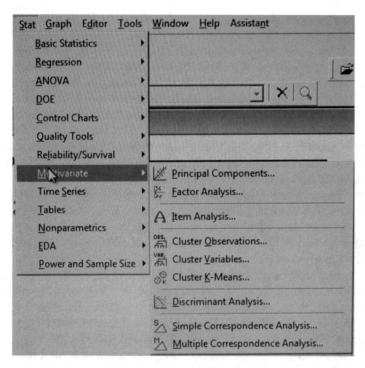

Fig. 3.9 Hovering over "Multivariate" displays a battery of useful analytic procedures, particularly principal component analysis, clustering, and discriminant analysis

"Stat:TimeSeries" contains a set of specific functions to analyze repeated measurements over time. The importance of these functions is that they allow an estimation of "autocorrelation" or "cyclic behavior," since in many circumstances the "next" measure is affected by the "previous" measure of the variable. A limiting aspect of most time series methods is that the intervals must be constant with no missing values. This is often a problem with retrospective data but should be straightforward when planning to measure something at regular intervals going forward (e.g., monthly readmissions, monthly wound infections), so it has an important place in quality improvement analyses. Although such variables might actually vary randomly over time, it is very possible that there are "trends" in the data that can be identified and addressed by understanding autocorrelation.

"Stat:Tables" contains a whole family of tests related to the chi-squared distribution. The chi-squared distribution is about COUNTS and applies to frequency data based on counting the number of events in specific categories. "Tally Individual Variables" counts the frequency of occurrence of each of the discrete values for any number of categorical variables in your dataset, and presents them as cell counts or cumulative (running) frequencies. "Cross-tabulation and Chi square" is a powerful tool that takes data in rows and columns, performs a cross-tabulation (the familiar two-by-two table as well as layered two-by-two tables), and then performs the variations on the chi-squared test. The term chi squared is applied to both a distribution and a test, but this menu applies specifically to the test (which is based on an underlying analysis of the distribution). We don't need to understand the specific applications of the distribution to be able to understand and apply the test. Suffice it to say that when count data can be expressed in one or more two-by-two tables, some test in the chi-squared family is appropriate. A peculiarity of the chi-squared test is that it is used on discrete data only BUT the underlying distribution function is actually continuous. This peculiarity is of no importance if the total number of counts is large, at least 100, where the traditional chi-squared test can be used. If the total count of all cells is less than 100, however, the peculiarity becomes important and must be corrected. Historically, this is accomplished by using a correction factor in the calculation called the Yates' (or continuity) correction. However, an alternative way to compensate is to perform the exact test which gives an exact probability calculated from the data. Traditionally this was recommended when any one cell in a two-by-two cell has a count less than 5. But modern computers can do the calculations quickly regardless of the counts, so the exact test can be performed routinely in place of chi squared. When there are layered two-by-two tables, each corresponding to a level of a third variable, the Mantel-Haenszel-Cochran test is performed. Both the exact and the Mantel-Haenszel-Cochran are found under (States:Cross-tabulationAndChiSquared:OtherTests).

"Stat:Nonparametrics" (Fig. 3.10) contains a family of statistical tests that are called nonparametric because they do not rely on estimated parameters and are thus distribution free. Traditional (parametric) statistical tests use a set of parameters (most commonly the mean and standard deviation), essentially disregarding the actual data, and perform the statistical analysis using only the parameters. This concept explains why adhering to the assumptions of the test (the characteristics of the parameters) is so important. Nonparametric tests do not make an assumption of distribution. They are particularly useful if initial analysis demonstrates that the data are not normally distributed, rather than searching for a suitable transform to normalize the data. The Mann-Whitney test is a nonparametric test comparable to an unpaired t-test; a Wilcoxon test to a paired t-test; and a Kruskal-Wallis test to a one way ANOVA. When a variable is not normally distributed, the simplest approach is to use a nonparametric test first. If the nonparametric test indicates that there IS a significant difference, it typically won't identify many of the other desirable statistics. Since, however, the hypothesis now changes from "is there a difference" to "since there is a difference, where is it," applying the parametric procedure allows the determination of the more detailed specifics available in many parametric methods.

"Stat:EDA" consists of a family of methods to conduct exploratory data analysis, allowing visual inspection of data to provide enhanced understanding, particularly of identifying outlier observations and analysis of residuals. It adds a visual component to the analysis of "descriptive statistics" as well as corroboration of the results of normality testing.

"Stat:PowerAndSampleSize" (Fig. 3.11) contains methods used in designing prospective experiments (determining the number of individuals required to provide a credible statistical analysis). We have already discussed "the likelihood of being

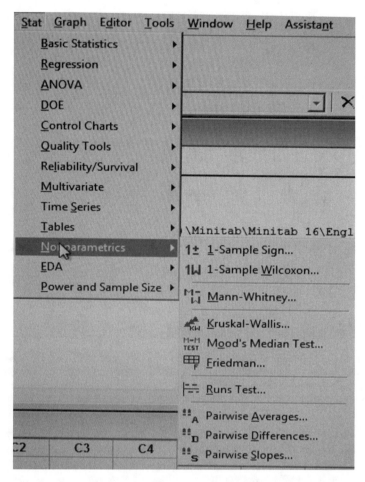

Fig. 3.10 Selecting "Non-parametrics" displays a full set of nonparametric statistical tests. The Wilcoxon and Mann-Whitney tests are comparable to paired and unpaired *t*-tests. The Kruskal-Wallis test is the nonparametric analogue to the one-way ANOVA, allowing comparison of multiple groups. The Friedman test is comparable to a two-way ANOVA

wrong" if we reject the null hypothesis (type 1 error) which is symbolized by the Greek letter alpha (α). Alpha is not affected by sample size except when it is "small" (<30). A type 2 error, which estimates how likely we are to be wrong if we do NOT reject the null hypothesis, beta (β), is very sensitive to sample size. Subtracting beta from "1" ($1-\beta$) is known as the power of the test. Sample size and power can be considered "opposite sides of the same coin" in that knowing one allows determination of the other. If we identify how willing we are to be wrong in NOT rejecting the null, we can estimate the number needed in each group. If we stipulate the number to be enrolled in each group, we can estimate the power. The family of statistical tests listed in the drop-down menu is amenable to power analysis. In retrospective data analysis, in which "n" is known, the power (already established but not known!) can

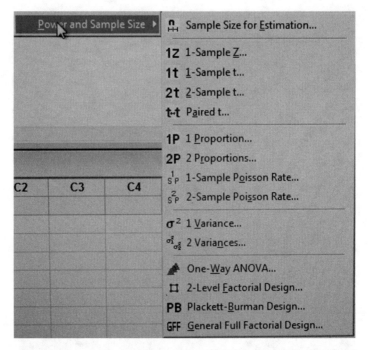

Fig. 3.11 Selecting "Power and Sample Size" opens a battery of procedures that assess "how good" a statistical test has performed. Power is equal to $(1 - \beta)$, where β is the probability of a type 2 error (saying there is no difference, when in fact there is). It is based on a given sample size. Alternatively, defining a "power" allows determination of the sample size required to achieve it

be estimated to provide an understanding of whether the results of having NOT rejected the null are likely to be repeatable. Understanding and knowing the power of the test are critically important in interpreting results that show NO DIFFERENCE (could the study actually have SHOWN a difference???).

We have specifically focused on methods using Minitab, but the same methods are available in all of the menu-driven statistical software packages. The actual command structure may differ slightly and the "look and feel" may not be the same, but the methods are essentially the same.

3.6 R, RExcel, and RCommander

As previously explained, "R" is a software environment that contains a very large collection of PACKAGES that each contains a set of related METHODS which were typically created by an expert in a specific analytical application. Some packages require the installation of other packages and most require the presence of a basic set of packages that are automatically loaded when "R" is initially downloaded. A more detailed introduction to "R" can be found in the Appendix.

CRAN (Comprehensive R Archive Network) is the formal term used to describe the whole "R" enterprise. It also serves as a very useful term in performing Google searches. By typing CRAN followed by one or two keywords describing what you are trying to do, you will get four or five very specific sites that should address the syntax, the contents, and at least one detailed review article. As explained previously, the hardest part of using "R" is that it's UNFORGIVING, so you will often return to the basic documents if you have not used a specific package for even a short while.

Instructions for installing "R" are found on the CRAN website (cran.r-project. org). Instructions for installing RExcel can be found on the Statconn website (rcom. univie.ac.at/download.html, then download). Since it is absolutely essential to follow both sets of instructions to the letter, read them both very carefully prior to downloading either software. In particular, on the "Download the latest version here" page, scroll down to the bottom of the section entitled "RExcel" and click on the hyperlink "Detailed instructions for installing can be found in our wiki." The most important tips to successfully installing and connecting the two software packages are found here. In addition, there is a specific package in "R" entitled "Rcmdr" that will import a saved Excel spreadsheet and allow menu commands for visualization and analysis. (NOTE: RExcel only works with 32-bit Excel, even on a 64-bit computer, but you can use Rcmdr with 64-bit Excel.)

Some additional tips about R and RExcel/RCommander:

- Neither is particularly user friendly, so be patient and be ACCURATE—if you enter something absolutely correctly, it will work.
- If you can write R-code, the "R" Console is easier to use—I still use it routinely for installing new packages, using the limited menu at the top (R:InstallPackages).
- R and RExcel are ABSOLUTELY case sensitive—if you err in case usage, either console (RConsole or RCommander) will tell you that the variable doesn't exist.
- The "enter" key is useless in RExcel but you only find out after you realize that nothing happened except advancing to the next line—use "Submit" each time.
- If you open both "R" and "RExcel" (actually RConsole and RCommander) keep in mind that they DON'T TALK TO EACH OTHER.

Once you have installed RExcel, you can find the command to start it both as an icon on the desktop (RExcel 2013 with R) and in the top menu bar in Excel (RExcel). Click either one and, after a pause, you will see RExcel pop up and then disappear. Now enter (Add-Ins:RExcel:Rcommander:WithExcelMenus:) and wait. After a pause, the RCommander window will ultimately appear and then disappear with an R icon appearing on the tray at the bottom of the screen. Remember the location of that icon! In addition, a row of menu items (toolbar) will have appeared at the top of the Excel spreadsheet, to the right of the blue "R." (Note: Alternatively you could have selected "with separate menus" and the menus would appear at the top of the RCommander window but if you are working in Excel, it is more convenient to have this toolbar in Excel.) Scroll through the menu options and familiarize yourself with the contents. If you use Excel as "home," most of your data manipulation can occur within Excel itself. However, once you have "put" your data into RExcel, changing the data within RExcel will require using the RExcel commands (Data:ActiveDataSet) in the toolbar.

You can also use this to change the names of variables within Excel, although it is preferable to make those changes in Excel prior to "putting" the dataset. An important concept when using R is to constantly be aware of where YOU are (in Excel, in RExcel, in R, etc.), since where your cursor is active determines what will happen.

RCommander can also be reached through RConsole (library(Rcmdr)). This approach requires importing the Excel file (Data:ImportData:fromExcelfile), but it has the advantage that there is a single R process working in the background that can be reached either by RConsole or RCommander.

The RExcel/RCommander toolbar is depicted in Fig. 3.4a and the Minitab screens in Fig. 3.4b. "Statistics" and "Graphs" are the most commonly used menu items in either RExcel or RCommander (Fig. 3.4b). If you are doing the initial work in Excel, "File" is rarely used. "Data" is only needed to modify data AFTER it has been "put" into R (Data:ManageVariablesInActiveDataset). "Statistics" (Fig. 3.12) contains many useful items. The top five items essentially repeat what was available in Excel:DataAnalysis. The bottom three (nonparametric tests, dimensional analysis, fit models) contain powerful tools for data analysis. Nonparametric tests include tests without distribution assumptions analogous to *t*-tests and ANOVA. Dimensional analysis contains tools which will be addressed in subsequent chapters.

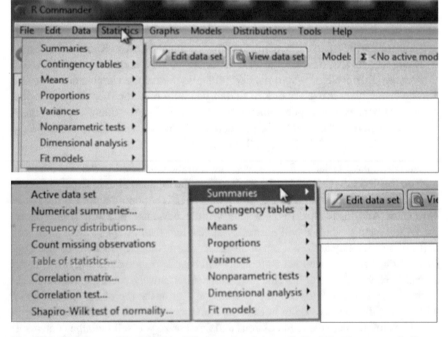

Fig. 3.12 Clicking on "Statistics" in RCommander shows a listing of options very similar to Minitab and hovering over "Summaries" shows a battery of summary statistics available using the menu. Note that only methods that are "applicable" to the selected data will be highlighted, while non-applicable methods will be faint

"Graphs" contains an incredible list of graphics options. The relevant options become bold when a dataframe is "put" into R. You should familiarize yourself with the graphics tools provided by RCommander. Although there is a "help" function in R and in RExcel, they aren't much help! Preferable is to Google CRAN and the item name (e.g., CRAN histogram) where thorough help is available.

"Models" contains advanced tools for evaluating models that are created with "fit models." You will find use for Akaike Information Criteria (AIC), stepwise model selection, best subset regression, numerical diagnostics, and graphs.

With this introduction, you are ready to "put" a dataset into RExcel or import it into Rcmdr. (If you prefer to enter your own commands, Chap. 1 in "The R Book" is helpful reading.) To "put" the dataframe into RExcel, highlight the entire range of data you wish to include, erring on the side of including rather than not including. Columns should be adjacent, so delete any extra columns. Right click within the highlighted area and select R:PutData:Dataframe. If your data are all numeric, you could choose Array, but Dataframe is preferable because it allows both numeric and non-numeric data. Although you will be prompted with a file name, change it to something short, simple, without capitals or symbols. Choosing "OK" will enter the name of your dataset into the menu toolbar. You can "put" more than one subset of data into RExcel, assigning a different name to each and switch between them in the "dataset" field, or you can use (Data:UseActiveDataset:SubsetActiveDataSet) to subset your data. To import a dataset into Rcmdr, click on Data:ImportData:fromExcel, enter a name for the file, and browse for the prepared Excel file.

3.7 Plotting

An important part of using any analytics software is being able to create graphs and plots. Each of the three software packages just addressed approaches plotting in a different way.

Excel is the most limited and often a bit "convoluted." Perhaps the most useful plotting function in Excel is the ability to create straight lines with the essential statistical information on a scatterplot (as previously described). Within "descriptive statistics," Excel has a function for creating histograms of data. It is awkward at best, as it requires user definition of the individual bins. However, it does allow creating unequal size bins or collapsing areas that contain no data, which might allow a more compact plot.

Minitab has a full menu of plotting functions under **Graph** (Fig. 3.13). **Scatterplot** is simple and straightforward—select two variables and the software does the rest. Of more use, perhaps, is a scatterplot matrix, under **Matrix Plot**, which creates a matrix of individual scatterplots, comprising every combination of variables that the user selects. Although the individual plots are small, they allow easy visualization of all of the paired relationships, which is particularly useful for determining if a distribution is unimodal or bimodal. Marginal Plot is an enhanced form of scatterplot, placing a histogram or boxplot along the upper and right margins of a scatterplot, which

Fig. 3.13 Selecting Graph in Minitab. Minitab has a full set of graphics options that are menu driven. In fact, Minitab is known for its ability to provide visualization. Most Minitab methods include an "Option" box to select what types of graphs should be displayed

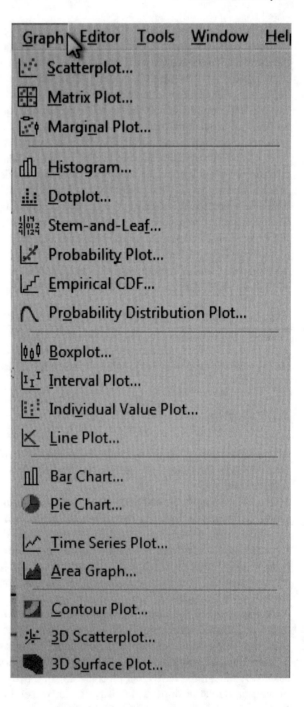

Fig. 3.14 Selecting Graph in RCommander displays a menu of graphic options very similar to Minitab

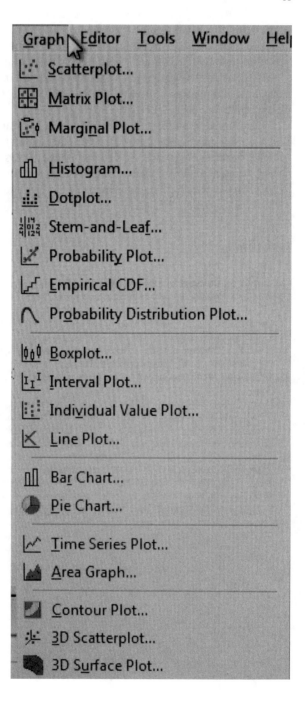

"aggregates" the relationships between the selected variables, allowing a sense of "joint distribution." **Histogram, Dotplot, and Stem-and-Leaf** plots are closely related methods of displaying the distribution of each variable, one variable at a time.

"R" repeats the plotting functions of Minitab (plus many more). "Plot" is a basic attribute of all R packages. In addition, RExcel and RCommander have menu-driven plotting functions (Fig. 3.14).

So in summary, no single software package is ideal for ALL of the aspects of analyzing data. A combination of packages that allows fluid movement among them (actually between Excel and each of the others) allows a comprehensive approach to analysis, facilitating understanding and improving the accuracy of predictive models. I can vouch for the combination of Excel, RExcel, and Minitab.

References

1. Dretzke BJ. Statistics with Microsoft Excel. 4th ed. Upper Saddle River: Prentice Hall; 2009.
2. Pace L. Beginning R, an introduction to statistical programming. New York: Apress; 2012. Distributed to the book trade worldwide by Springer Science + Business Media.
3. Quirk TJ, Horton H, Quirk M. Excel 2010 for biological and life sciences statistics a guide to solving practical problems. New York, NY: Springer; 2013.
4. Quirk TJ, Cummings S. Excel 2010 for health services management statistics: a guide to solving practical problems. Cham: Springer; 2014.
5. Schmuller J. Statistical analysis with Excel for dummies. 2nd ed. Hoboken: John Wiley & Sons, Inc; 2009.
6. Newton I. Minitab Cookbook. Birmingham: Packt Publishing; 2014.
7. Crawley MJ. The R book, vol. xxiv. 2nd ed. Chichester: Wiley; 2013. 1051 pages.
8. Crawley MJ. Statistics: an introduction using R. 2nd ed. Hoboken: Wiley; 2014.
9. Dalgaard P. Introductory statistics with R (SpringerLink). 2nd ed. New York: Springer; 2008.
10. Schumacker RE, Tomek S. Understanding statistics using R. New York, NY: Springer; 2013.
11. Spector P. Data manipulation with R (SpringerLink). New York: Springer; 2008.
12. Teetor P, Loukides MK. R cookbook. 1st ed. Beijing: O'Reilly; 2011.
13. Heiberger RM, Neuwirth E. R through Excel a spreadsheet interface for statistics, data analysis, and graphics (SpringerLink). New York: Springer; 2009.

Chapter 4
Measurement and Uncertainty

Scenario

Ron Silverman is a medical oncologist with an interest in managing recurrent colorectal cancer. He read an article about statistical trend analysis and thought that it might be interesting to examine a potential model for tracking CEA levels in patients who undergo potentially curative resection of high-risk lesions. He starts measuring CEA monthly in a large cohort of patients, starting 3 months after surgery. He takes the first six levels and determines for each patient the month-to-month variability of levels and the amount of increase that should trigger a suspicion of recurrence. He is amazed at the ability to identify recurrence many months before any of the imaging tests suggest it. In fact, he realizes that by understanding the "stochastic variability" of the CEA levels in individual patients, even increases within the reported normal range can be indicative. He sets out to develop an NIH grant proposal (**measurement, stochastic variability, control limits**).

4.1 The Stochastic Nature of Data

When looking at a number, 14.6 for example, it is easy to believe that the value is actually 14.6. In fact, it could have been 14.5 or 14.7 or, less likely, 14.4 or 14.8. In addition, measuring it a second time will usually give a slightly different result than the first. All measurement has uncertainty. Some of the uncertainty is due to actual error in the measurements (instrumental error or systematic error), but much is due to random variability (**stochasticity**). Unfortunately, medicine is usually taught as "deterministic" (if this, then that), and we tend to overlook the role of randomness and error.

© Springer International Publishing Switzerland 2016

P.J. Fabri, *Measurement and Analysis in Transforming Healthcare Delivery*,
DOI 10.1007/978-3-319-40812-5_4

4.1.1   The Distribution Functions of Data

Consider a single measurement in a single patient. That value is actually a member
of a family of possible measurements that follow what is called a "**probability distribution function**" **or** "**pdf**" [1]. When you perform multiple measurements, that
pdf starts to become visible. With repeated measurements over time, or with multiple patients, that variability (within measurements, between measurements, within
subjects, between subjects) results in a different and more complex "joint" pdf. The
most widely known pdf is the **normal distribution**—Gaussian, bell shaped
(Fig. 4.1), but there are many other distributions of measurements important to medicine: measurements of time typically follow an exponential distribution, waiting
time a variant called a gamma function, failure rates another variant known as the
Weibull, counts a Poisson distribution, ratios of two variables a Cauchy distribution,
and many laboratory results lognormal. While it is tempting to ignore this and
assume that everything "fits" a normal distribution, such an approach introduces a
very real (and unknown!) level of error in analysis and modeling because the
assumptions of the method or model are not being met [1]. A rough rule of thumb
in considering normality is to ask if a result as much lower than the normal or average as the highest result realistically imaginable is actually possible. For example,

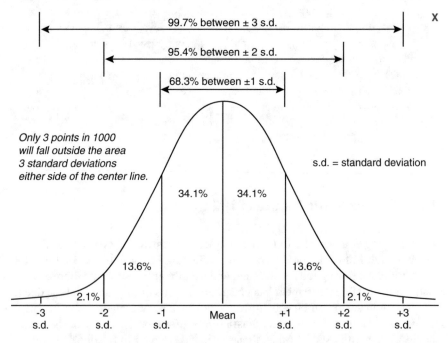

Fig. 4.1   The "normal curve" is a mathematical construct and, as such, does not actually represent
"reality." Some data (particularly related to biology and agriculture) can be fairly represented by
the normal distribution, but many others cannot, which results in erroneous conclusions. Many
distributions in healthcare have a long tail to the right. Note that when there is a long tail to the
right, the convention of two standard deviations representing the 95 % upper limit would not actually represent 95 %

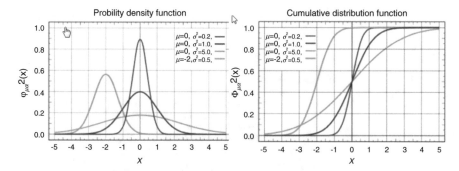

Fig. 4.2 The probability distribution function (on the *left*) displays the frequency occurring at each level of data. When the data are discrete, it is known as a probability MASS function. When the frequency accumulates, starting from the left, the cumulative distribution function displays the % included up to that level. (1−CDF) represents the right side of the curve, the % NOT INCLUDED. Note how each curve changes with different values for the mean (μ) and variance (σ^2)

if a "normal" plasma amylase level is 40–140 U/L, could I expect to have a result equally smaller as larger. Recognizing that I have seen results over 3000, it is immediately apparent that the answer is no. If the answer is no, then it is probably not a normal distribution and a search for a more appropriate distribution would be helpful. The normal (Gaussian) distribution is symmetrical, bell shaped, and characterized by two parameters, the mean (central tendency) and the standard deviation (dispersion) (Fig. 4.2). It has a counterpart **cumulative distribution function (cdf)** that "accumulates" a probability sum, starting at the left side of the graph and "accumulating" the area under the curve. The resulting cdf starts at 0 % and, moving to the right, progressively increases until 100 % is reached, having created a "sigmoidal curve." Visualizing the pdf is helpful because it graphically depicts the shape of the distribution curve. Looking at the cdf, picking a value of the variable on the *x*-axis and locating it on the cumulative distribution curve allow identification of the percentile that that value represents (or alternatively identifying a percentile on the *y*-axis defines the corresponding value on the *x*-axis). The points corresponding to 25, 50, 75, and 100 % are the 1st, 2nd, 3rd, and 4th quartiles.

4.1.2   *Understanding Uncertainty Requires Understanding DIKW*

Moving from a set of data to the ability to mindfully use the data involves a series of processes (data:information:knowledge:wisdom—Fig. 4.3). While moving through an analysis, it is important to keep in mind where in that series you are and where in that series you need to be next. Knowing only, for example, that the blood glucose is 175 mg/dl often leads to a single, standardized approach to management. Putting the data into a context (a 75-year-old postoperative patient in the ICU receiving corticosteroids and inotropic agents) and understanding the actual distributions of blood glucose for the population in consideration (extended tail to the right) often result in a different

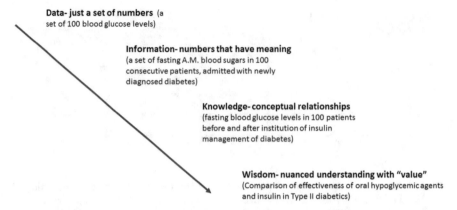

Fig. 4.3 The DIKW hierarchy (again), showing its application to the measurement of blood glucose levels

clinical approach. A visual demonstration of this can be created easily in a modern electronic medical record by graphing the blood glucose levels obtained in the hospital laboratory for a particular patient and the multiple fingerstick glucose measurements performed at the bedside in the same graph. Some of the corresponding results are similar but often they aren't, differing by 30, 50, or even 100 mg/dl. The same can be seen with blood pressure in the ICU: arterial line pressure and cuff pressure. It is easy to assume that they are measuring the same thing, but a moment's thought will confirm that they are actually measuring related but VERY DIFFERENT physical properties. The arterial line is measuring a transduced pressure wave (not flow!) while the cuff is using the sound or vibration produced by turbulent flow. Although they often produce similar measurements, there is no reason why they MUST. Understanding the sources of the data and the processes involved in advancing from information into knowledge/ wisdom will enhance the understanding of uncertainty and variability. And there are other sources of error or variation that need to be understood.

Systematic error is the "cousin" of random variability. Measuring the same thing over and over again yields random variation. Using an erroneous measuring device results in systematic error, as would incorrect use of a "true" measuring device, as does using two different individuals to measure. ALL measurements are "off" by a certain amount. Random error contributes to variance (dispersion), while systematic error contributes to bias (shift).

4.2   Databases, Datasets, and Dataframes

A **database** is a structured collection of data in a computer. While a database may consist exclusively of data units that could be collected on a Rolodex (known as a flat-file), most modern databases consist of a network of interrelated tables, connected by common links (known as relational). This is more efficient because it avoids the need to repeatedly enter redundant information (linking several laboratory test results by a patient ID number versus entering name, address, etc. repeatedly for each lab test). Typically, the structure of a database was created to facilitate data entry, using a data-entry template, and data presentation, using a query template. Each unit of data entered would be "directed" to a different table in the database, and later re-extracted and reassembled into a query report. The entry report looks like a simple set of rows and columns as does the query report. The actual structure of the database can be conceptualized as a network of individual tables (e.g., demographic information, dates of visits, laboratory results) interconnected by a large number of connecting lines known as joins. The entire database can often not be presented in a spreadsheet, because although "linked" they don't exactly "match": there is likely more than one lab visit or lab result per visit and more than one visit per patient. This can be resolved with a "query" that "asks" the database engine to assemble a specific spreadsheet. A **dataset** has thus been extracted from a database. If the dataset consists only of numeric entries and their variable names, it represents an **array**, but often a dataset also contains non-numeric data. The term to describe a structured collection of <u>different types of data</u> in "R" and other similar environments is a **dataframe**.

To create a predictive model to evaluate/predict readmissions to the hospital after discharge for congestive heart failure, first find all of the appropriate databases, create linkages between the databases to associate the records, and conduct a query. This would produce a dataset that could be imported into Excel as a spreadsheet, allowing assessing, visualizing, and analyzing the data to create models.

4.3 Missing Values

Many analytical methods either will not work at all or will provide erroneous answers if there are missing values. Others are more "robust" to missing values. For the less "robust" methods, it is imperative that the missing values are "replaced." But how? There are numerous approaches to "filling in" missing values (some simple and some quite complex). A simple but effective approach is to replace a missing value with the average value for the column. This won't change the overall mean for the column and, if "n" is of reasonable size, it won't change the standard deviation either. Functionally it is as if nothing "new" has been added to the data, yet it would allow the method to "work." For a variable that is clearly not normally distributed, the median can be used in a similar way, or the variable can be transformed and the missing value replaced by the mean of the newly transformed column. Keep in mind that the goal is to allow the method to proceed without changing the original data. However, it is important to recognize how many missing values exist both by column and by row. If values are missing in a specific column, adding a large number of "means" won't change the mean but it will begin to affect the standard deviation. If there are multiple missing values by row, it may be preferable to delete the row(s) entirely if sufficient rows will remain in the dataset. If you know that the data distribution for a column of data is NOT normal, using the median might be preferable. A more complicated approach is to "interpolate" values based on other columns of data, but this is rarely necessary and much more difficult.

4.4   Probability, Likelihood, and Odds

The terms **probability** and **likelihood** are often used interchangeably, but in the strictest sense, they have different meanings. "Probability" actually exists—it is a known quantity, usually based on a scientific principle, such as flipping a coin has a 50% probability of heads, and can be applied to the occurrence of an event. "Likelihood" is a measured quantity from data, not scientifically defined, such as the likelihood of appendicitis. A coin could be flipped 100 times to determine if the likelihood of heads matches the mathematical probability of heads (in other words, is the coin fair?). Statistical methods are often based on a likelihood function [$L(x)$], which is "maximized" using **optimization** methods to determine the parameters of a defined distribution (such as Gaussian) for a set of data (collectively referred to as maximum likelihood estimate—MLE). A ratio of estimated likelihoods of two different models (maximum likelihood ratio) can be used and, traditionally, the logarithm is used to facilitate the math resulting in the **log-likelihood ratio**. **Odds** is simply the ratio of the probability or likelihood of YES divided by the probability or likelihood of NO. Since $P(no) = 1 - P(yes)$, odds is typically expressed as $O = P(yes)/(1 - P(yes))$ or $x/(1 - x)$. Stated another way, seeing "$x/(1 - x)$" should suggest that it is odds. Conversely, through simple algebra, if O = the observed , then $P(yes) = Odds/(1 + Odds)$. Seeing an equation resembling $z/(1 + z)$ should identify a probability or likelihood. Additionally, a ratio of two different odds is simply $[P(x)/(1 - P(x)]/[P(y)/(1 - P(y)]$. These relationships will become very important when we begin creating analytical models. What is the easiest way to think of these concepts—probability/likelihood versus odds? Much as we can understand combinations of hemoglobin and hematocrit—two different ways to express essentially the same concept. Which value do we use clinically? The one we have at hand, usually hemoglobin in modern times. With only a hematocrit value, and little effort, we can convert back to hemoglobin by using an assumed value of the MCHC (typically about 33), so hemoglobin is roughly 1/3 of the hematocrit. So too with probability and odds. More practically, probability/likelihood is intuitively understandable, while odds is how the math is done.

4.5   Logit and Logistic

These terms are very often used in statistics and modeling but are usually "foreign" to clinicians. In years gone by, before computers, taking a logarithm was commonly performed (from tables or using slide rules) because adding a series of logarithms was easier than multiplying a series of large numbers by hand. Specific names were given to the logarithms of common entities. Taking the log of $(1/(1 - x))$ (the log-odds) is called **logit(x)**. Conversely, the log of $y/(1 + y)$ (the log-probability) is the **logistic(y)**. It can be very confusing when these terms are first confronted in equations, which is easily remedied by recalling that they are simply the logarithms of common entities.

4.6 Induction Versus Deduction

In a designed experiment, in which the measurements and the statistical approach have been defined in advance and the data actually collected and entered by the investigator, it is possible to arrive at a logical answer based on the "facts." This is an example of **deduction**. To the question "what is two plus two," there is only a single answer. However, when data have been collected by someone else, typically for a very different purpose, and are now being examined retrospectively to identify relationships, the thought processes are quite different—**induction**. Now the question is "if the answer is four, what two numbers were used." Immediately $2+2$ and $3+1$ come to mind. But alternatively it could be $-3000+3004$ or an infinite number of other combinations, some of which are more likely based on the context. In this case, it is not possible to arrive at a definite answer, just a more likely one. As physicians, we are taught to analyze data as if there is a single, correct (deductive) conclusion. But in fact that is rarely the case. For example, other diseases can be associated with the same abnormal laboratory tests, such as the lupus antigen.

Another example is sensitivity versus predictive value. Medical students memorize the concepts of sensitivity and specificity in order to pass multiple-choice exams. In clinical practice, these concepts are rarely addressed—an abnormal test automatically MEANS disease. But in fact, laboratory test results are used INDUCTIVELY, which requires an understanding of the uncertainty of induction. A helpful way to incorporate these concepts into practice is to recognize both sensitivity and the predictive value of a positive test and specificity and the predictive value of a negative test. Sensitivity is a **conditional probability**—in this case the likelihood of a positive test result GIVEN the presence of disease—using notation, $P(+|D)$. Specificity, similarly, is the likelihood of a negative test GIVEN the absence of disease—$P(-|N)$. Clinicians don't typically see patients with known disease and perform tests to see if the tests are abnormal. Rather we see a single patient while considering a single laboratory result. The actual question is what is the likelihood of disease GIVEN an abnormal test result (known as the **predictive value of a positive test**)—$P(D|+)$, or alternatively what is the likelihood of no disease GIVEN a normal test result (the **predictive value of a negative test**)—$P(N|-)$. These latter concepts rely on the actual likelihood of the disease and are "inductive" because other diseases might also be associated with the same abnormal test result (both acute liver disease and myocardial infarction can elevate transaminase levels and an anterior compartment syndrome can increase CPK). Accepting the fact that the laboratory tests currently offered by an accredited laboratory have sufficient sensitivity and specificity to be clinically useful, then the predictive values are influenced by the likelihood of the disease and the likelihood of a positive (or negative) test result, not the "given" sensitivity of the test. This concept is an application of **Bayes' theorem** and is considered in more detail later. At this point, what is important is to recognize that most of clinical medicine is NOT deductive, but rather inductive, inferred, and requires a consideration of alternative explanations based on likelihoods—another example of the uncertainty of medicine. Context is usually as important as the data!

4.7   Bias

In a social context, bias is often thought of negatively, as in discrimination or unfairness. In statistics, bias has a definite but neutral meaning. Bias is the systematic difference between what is observed and what is expected. In high school, we learned how to graph the equation for a straight line ($y = ax + b$) with the line crossing the y-axis at the y-intercept. In analytics, the y-intercept is the **bias** of a metric and, rather than just a single point on the y-axis, it is a "floor" or "baseline" that extends all the way across the x–y graph, with each data point being displaced up (or down) by the bias.

This means that ALL of the measurements are offset, either up or down, by a fixed amount (although it is also possible that the amount varies in a proportionate way). It may help to think of it this way—in a perfect world, if x equals zero, then y should theoretically be zero as well. In the real world it often isn't, and the measurements are offset by some amount. This is NOT random error or inconsistent use of a measuring device. It is a systematic and consistent deviation. It COULD be due to a faulty measuring device (a 12.5 in foot ruler; a scale that shows two pounds of weight while empty) or it could be due to a systematic difference in the circumstances of a measurement (barometric pressure measured on top of a mountain). Bias exists commonly in data and must be understood rather than ignored. Consideration should also be given to the possibility that the bias might NOT be constant, but varies in a systematic way as x increases (probably recognized in a correlation matrix and subsequently identified by a method known as ANCOVA, analysis of covariance), separately from the measurement of interest (for example measuring bone density over time to assess a treatment effect requires understanding the underlying variation in bone density simply due to age). This concept becomes even more bewildering when we move from physical measurements to areas such as cognitive or psychological metrics.

4.8   Residuals

The term **residual** is another expression of the mathematical difference between each value in a set of values and the expectation for that value (a common expected value is given by the mean). If there is more than one expected value, there can be more than one residual in a single analysis.

For example, in a column of entries for a variable, subtracting the mean for the column from each of the entries results in a column of residuals. These same residuals, when squared to produce only positive values (sum of squared residuals) and divided by the degrees of freedom—dof (typically $n-1$)—produce the variance for that column [$\sigma^2 = \Sigma(y - \hat{y})^2/(n-1)$]. But that total sum of squared residuals can also be subdivided (or **partitioned**) when constructing a linear model (as we shall see later) into a component due to a relationship (called the sum of squared residuals due to regression—SSR) and a component due to random variability (called the sum of squared residuals due to error—SSE). When dealing with "residuals," focus on which meaning of residuals is being addressed. Analysis of variance (ANOVA), analysis of covariance (ANCOVA), and linear regression are all based on residuals.

Graphing residuals in various formats highlights the importance of looking at the structure and variation of the residuals to better understand a dataset (Fig. 4.4). Calculating the individual residuals results in a number of important measures of variability.

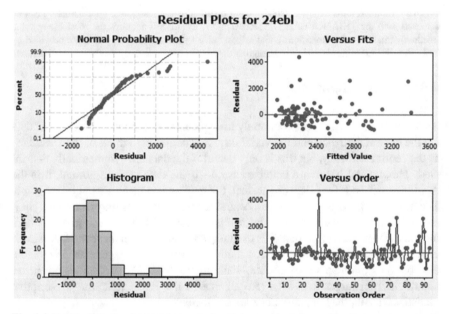

Fig. 4.4 Residual plots—determining and visualizing residuals is a critically important step in analysis. Residuals are the difference between the actual data and some form of expected value. These four plots (from a model to predict perioperative blood loss—ebl) are typical and assess four different aspects of the distribution of the residuals $(y - \hat{y})$: the "normal probability plot" shows how the actual residuals (*red dots*) deviate from the expected residuals if it were a normal distribution—the deviation suggests non-normality; "versus fits" shows that the residuals appear larger for smaller values of x—an indicator of probable non-normality; "histogram" shows the actual frequency distribution of the residuals—a long tail to the right (skew) suggesting non-normality; "versus order" shows larger residuals to the right, representing later data points, suggesting a deterioration of a process or tool over time—once again non-normality. It is important not to confuse these as each approach to residuals examines a different characteristic of the data

- An easy way to visualize the shape of a distribution of numbers
- Requires an estimation of:
  - (a) lowest likely level (maximum)
  - (b) highest likely level (minimum)
  - (c) most likely level (mode)

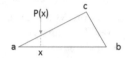

$$P(x)= \begin{cases} 0, & x < a \\ \dfrac{2(x-a)}{(b-a)(c-a)}, & a \leq x \leq c \\ \dfrac{2(b-x)}{(b-a)(b-c)}, & c \leq x \leq b \\ 0, & x > b \end{cases}$$

Fig. 4.5 Although tools exist to identify actual distributions, a reasonable approximation can be achieved with the TRIANGULAR DISTRIBUTION, which only requires the most likely value (median), smallest value (minimum), and largest value (maximum), all of which are provided by basic statistics in most software. The triangular distribution is particularly useful for small datasets

4.9   Central Tendency

As mentioned, the two most commonly used parameters for a variable or set of data are the central tendency and the variability. It is common to think of the "average" as the central tendency, but this is only useful if the data are symmetrically distributed. The median is often a better measure—if the data are non-normal, it is the "middlemost" and if the data are normal, the median and mean should be the same. The mode is a third way to estimate central tendency, but it is only usable for "unimodal" data or in generating an empirical **triangular distribution** (Fig. 4.5), where the **most likely value** (the mode) is used together with the smallest and largest values to create a pdf. The triangular distribution is a useful way to generate a workable distribution from a small set of data, while more "formal" distributions are better identified from larger data sets. (Recall that in the Excel function "Descriptive Statistics," mean, median, and mode are all displayed.)

4.10   Variability

The "width" of a distribution can be estimated from a parameter, the variance, or its square root, the standard deviation. Taking the square root of the variance returns the process to the original units of measure and estimates the variability of individual values. Dividing the standard deviation by the square root of "n" estimates the standard error (variability) of the mean—how much the MEAN varies as opposed to individual values. Thought of another way, the variance is the sum of squared residuals of a set of data divided by the number of degrees of freedom, so it's the adjusted average squared residual (making the standard deviation essentially the average residual!). When the median is used, however, the **interquartile range (IQR)** is a more useful estimator of width (as is typically used in boxplots). The IQR is the difference in values between the point representing the 75th percentile (third quartile) and the 25th percentile (first quartile). It "trims" off the tails, focusing on the central portion of the distribution. So a nonparametric counterpart to the mean and standard deviation is the median and IQR. Note that the variance and standard deviation can be calculated regardless of the underlying distribution—its meaning differs, but it can still be estimated. If the data are "normal," the standard deviation is a parameter representing the width of the representative normal distribution and the parameters can be used in place of the actual data. But if the data are NOT normal, then the standard deviation is just a calculated value, which can be compared to another standard deviation but not used in place of the actual data! In use, determining the ratio of variances between/among different categories of the same measurement (e.g., males/females) can be used to assess whether the variances are equal (**F-test**). This knowledge influences the choice of analytical method—some "require" equal variances while others are more robust to unequal variance. A useful "rule of thumb" is if the larger variance is less than twice the smaller, they are "close enough." Another way to look at variance is to assess how it changes as a function of some other measure, the variance of "y" as "x" changes, the variance as a function of time, etc. Since the variance is directly calculated from the residuals, the various graphic and mathematical methods to examine residuals are the most useful and practical way to understand these nuances of variance. When the variance is uniform across a range, the term **homoscedastic** is used; **heteroscedastic** means nonuniform, frequently increasing variance as the variable increases.

4.11 Centering and Standardizing

Centering of the elements of a variable is accomplished by subtracting the mean from each element. Recall that this is also the approach to determine residuals. More generally, centering produces a measure of distance from a reference point. This simplifies the interpretation in regression, by shifting everything "to the left," placing the location of the y-intercept (bias) in the center of the range of data rather than at the far left end where $x=0$ (often not actually included in the dataset). More importantly, centering does not change the analytical model (coefficients remain the same) except by shifting the intercept. In addition, centering is occasionally a required preliminary to other analysis (such as PCA). **Standardizing** takes centering one step further. It is the process of converting several variables of very different magnitude into a common scale (neutralizing the 3000-pound gorilla, so to speak). By subtracting the mean for a variable and dividing by the standard deviation, the data are converted into z-scores, all with a mean$=0$ and a standard deviation$=1$. This "balances" the contributions of large and small variables (shoe size and annual income). Like centering, standardizing does not change the relationships among the coefficients, but it does change their apparent magnitudes.

4.12   Homogeneity of Variances

Variance is the mathematical determination of the average squared residual. In analyzing/comparing two or more subsets of data, most methods estimate a common value for variance/standard deviation (based on assuming the null of no difference) often called "pooled." The underlying assumption is that if the subsets were obtained from the same population, they should have the same underlying variance/standard deviation, resulting in a more "robust" estimate. However, when a variance is being partitioned into components, as in the many forms of ANOVA, the underlying distributions may NOT be the same, and non-equality (non-homogeneity, heteroscedasticity) can influence the analysis to some <u>unknown</u> degree. Some methods are more susceptible (less robust) to non-homogeneity than others (more robust). Purists would say that since I don't know exactly how wrong I will be, I will either transform my data to produce more homogeneous variances or I will use analytical methods that are not dependent on parameters. Since there are no "variance police" or "variance judges," it is left to the analyst to make the determination and, since it is easier to assume that it doesn't matter, that is often selected. But this adds an unknown element of uncertainty and potential error in the interpretation.

4.13   Quantile (QQ) and Other Useful Plots

Minitab, R, and most other analytics software provide a number of additional plotting functions that provide alternative ways or combined ways to look at the data (Fig. 4.6). Their purpose is to provide different ways to visualize concepts. More detailed descriptions of each of these plots, with examples, can be found in the "help" function of the analytics software, also providing the specifics of how to use the function in that software.

The **QQ plot** shows the corresponding "rankings" (using the four quartiles for each variable, as opposed to the actual values) of a pair of variables, allowing a visual estimation of how they vary in relation to each other (joint distribution), while minimizing the importance of the magnitudes of the differences. A **scatterplot matrix** or matrix plot displays a full set of pairs of data and often includes histograms or pdfs of the individual variables. It is the most familiar, and represents the x–y location of each data point as a dot on the x–y graph. A **marginal plot** adds the histograms of the variables along the margins of a scatterplot, essentially decomposing the joint distribution back into its components. An **empirical CDF** creates the cumulative distribution function from the actual data, allowing visual assessment of where most of the variability in a distribution occurs. **Individual distribution plots** of different potential distributions can be generated from an entered set of

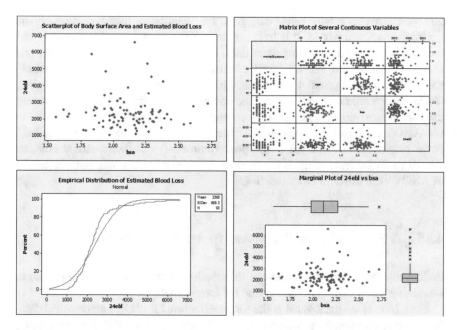

Fig. 4.6 Visualizing data is important, as the human eye can "see" things that the mind may not recognize. *Upper left*—SCATTERPLOT of two variables (bivariate plot); *upper right*—SCATTERPLOT MATRIX showing all selected variables, pairwise; *lower left*—empirical distribution showing the actual cumulative frequency (*red*) and the expected cumulative frequency if the data were normally distributed (*blue*), allowing a visual assessment of the distribution of residuals; *bottom right*—MARGINAL PLOT which augments the scatterplot by including boxplots on the upper and right margins for each variable, allowing comparison of the univariate distributions and the joint relationship

parameters and displayed graphically to visualize what a distribution with specified parameters looks like. **Boxplots** visualize the distribution of the data vertically, highlighting the median as well as the first and third quartiles (the IQR). In addition, they show the datapoints in the "tails" above and below the IQR as well as those values that are "extreme outliers" as asterisks.

4.14   Likert Scales and Likert Plots

Survey data often use rating scales (frequently called Likert scales, pronounced "lick-ert") with a fixed number (typically five to ten) of choices. A common example is strongly disagree (1), disagree (2), neutral (3), agree (4), and disagree (5). Focusing on the names of the variables makes it obvious that these are inexact measures with undefined interval distances. Replacing the names with numbers, however, provides a false sense that these are quantitative measures, appropriate for mathematical analysis. It is tempting to utilize parametric statistical tests and quantitative plots in analyzing such data. But rating scales are <u>ordinal data</u> and should be visualized and analyzed as such. Nonparametric tests appropriately address the data as ordinal. Likert plots, which are more properly called **diverging, stacked bar charts**, visually depict the counts of the individual choices in a way that facilitates understanding and comparison. Although it is common to see ANOVA applied to Likert-based data, the results should be "questioned." If the original data display a single peak (unimodal) with symmetrical tails, an ANOVA may be reasonable. If the data are bimodal or with a long tail, the results of ANOVA are likely to be misleading.

4.15   A Summary for Preparing to Analyze a Dataset

Pulling together this large amount of information allows mapping an approach to examining a new dataset in preparation for formal analysis.

First, look at the data. What is the format/structure? If it's in a hierarchical database, can it be broken up into distinct and logical parts, or will it require doing individual queries to create meaningful spreadsheets?

Put the data into spreadsheet form with variable names in the top row of columns, using simple, lower case variable names without symbols or punctuation.

After scanning over the entire dataset visually, use Conditional Formatting to identify empty cells.

Perform Descriptive Statistics in Excel, carefully assessing the maximum and minimum (to identify potential outliers or errors), the similarity of the mean and mode, skewness, and kurtosis. Look across the table of results and examine the relationship of the variances—are they similar? Identify the most likely outcome variables and move them to the right side of the dataset. If the descriptive statistics suggest that something in the data is awry, (an unrealistic high outlier, for example) more specific conditional formatting will find the culprit data entries.

Perform a correlation matrix and a correlation matrix plot of only the input variables. Are there any individual input correlations that are less than 0.10 or greater than 0.90? Look carefully at the correlation plot matrix. Which variables are asymmetrical or show wide variability? Which variables demonstrate an obvious, visual relationship, suggesting collinearity.

Repeat the correlation matrix and plot using <u>all</u> of the variables, input and output. Are the potential outcome variables correlated? Which of the input variables have less than 0.10 correlation with the outcome variables. In the correlation plot matrix which variables are asymmetrical or show wide variability?

Create boxplots of all of the individual variables—are they symmetrical or are there asymmetric outliers? Perform normality tests on any suspect variables. For those variables that are not normally distributed, are they visually symmetric. If asymmetrical, use Individual Distribution Identification to evaluate different transformations and their effects on normality.

Look at the residual plots of the transformations to see if the residuals are evenly distributed or increase at the ends or in the middle of the standardized residual plots. Are any of the variables so much larger (or smaller) than the others that standardization will bring them into a more uniform size range?

Perform scatterplots of individual input variables and outcome variables and visually assess the shape of the relationship (linear or nonlinear).

The more time spent in understanding the data and the relationships in the data, the better the subsequent models will be. A variable or residual that is visually asymmetric may substantially influence the usefulness of a model. Marked differences in the magnitude of variables could result in a model that is overwhelmed by the larger variable. An "apparent" relationship between two variables that doesn't make any logical sense could be spurious and should be viewed with caution—not ignored, just suspect.

Reference

1. Hand DJ. Statistics and the theory of measurement. J R Stat Soc Ser A. 1996;150(3):445–92.

Part II
Applying a Scientific Approach to Data Analysis

Chapter 5
Mathematical and Statistical Concepts in Data Analysis

Scenario

Ken Matsumoto and Ajit Raji are coninvestigators in a study to analyze an existing database to determine factors that influence the development of post-operative wound infections. The database has over 125 data fields. Ken feels strongly that as many variables as possible should be included in the model, to avoid "losing data." Ajit, however, explains to him that the simplest model with the smallest number of variables that provides the optimum ability to predict is preferable to a model with a larger number of variables. He calls this the "bias-variance trade-off," because adding more variables after the model is "tight" only increases the amount of variability.

5.1 A Brief Introduction to Mathematics

After a thorough preliminary analysis of the data and visualization of the distributions and relationships, a more quantitative and statistical approach can proceed. Such an approach requires an understanding of more advanced mathematical and statistical concepts, which will be addressed in Part 2. This review presents the information in a manner that should make sense to a physician with only the math and sciences learned in college and medical school. Readers who are interested in more depth of detail should consult the references.

© Springer International Publishing Switzerland 2016
P.J. Fabri, *Measurement and Analysis in Transforming Healthcare Delivery*,
DOI 10.1007/978-3-319-40812-5_5

5.2   Vectors and Matrices

The concept of vectors and matrices, introduced earlier, is fundamental to analytics. Because this is a "foreign concept," I will briefly repeat it. Most simply, a vector (usually described as an arrow into space with length and direction) is actually just a collection of related data that makes sense, which can be plotted on a graph with an arrow drawn from the origin. In a spreadsheet of aggregated hospital laboratory values for a specific day and time, a single column of blood glucose levels is a vector. A single row containing all laboratory values for a patient on a particular morning is also a vector. Combining a set of column vectors (or row vectors) together (that make sense) produces a matrix. Note that if you create a matrix from a set of columns it is the same matrix that you would create with the corresponding set of rows. The advantage of using vectors and matrices (as opposed to individual data points) is that the mathematics are more efficient and computers can do it faster. It is also a concise way to keep things orderly.

Vector and matrix mathematics are very analogous to traditional mathematics with a few important distinctions:

Addition and subtraction require that the elements have the same dimensions.
Multiplication is order-specific meaning that you can multiply on the left or multiply on the right and each way will give a different answer.
Division is not defined but multiplication by the inverse is.
Vectors can be reoriented in space (rotation and scaling).
Matrices can both transform and be transformed by other vectors and matrices (transformation accomplishes rotation, scaling, and skewing but moving a vector or matrix from one place to another without transforming it does not alter it).
Translating (moving a vector from one place to another) is called an "affine" function, and doesn't change anything (think affinity).
Transposing a vector or matrix interchanges the row space and the column space.
A special matrix, a square matrix with ones on the diagonal and zeros elsewhere, is known as the identity matrix and is basically a multidimensional "1."
Multiplying a matrix by its inverse, either on the left or on the right, yields the identity matrix of the same dimension.

Understanding some notation is essential:

A lower case variable in bold or with a straight line over it is a vector.
A bold capital variable is a matrix.
Placing a "-1" exponent after the symbol for a vector or matrix represents the inverse.
Placing a "t" exponent or an apostrophe (')after the symbol for a vector or matrix represents the transpose (exchanging rows and columns).
An upside-down A ($\forall$) means that the preceding statement applies "for all."
{ } means "is in the set."
Syntax commands in analytical software are generally set off with simple parentheses.

While there are many more symbols used in textbooks, these are the important ones for our purposes.

5.3   Arrays and Data Frames

It is fairly straightforward to think of a column of numbers in a spreadsheet as a vector representing many examples of a variable. Similarly, a row within a spreadsheet representing a single patient can also be thought of as a "patient vector." Combining the two together means that the actual spreadsheet can be thought of as a very large matrix, that is, if it only includes <u>numerical entries</u> and only has <u>two dimensions</u>. Adding a third (or more) dimension exceeds our ability to visualize and so often creates confusion. A "matrix-like" structure with more than two dimensions is known as an array, and it still only contains numerical entries. The term data frame has been coined to allow the inclusion of non-numerical variables (nominal, ordinal). Using "data frames" keys the software to the possibility of manipulations on non-numeric variables. It is easy to understand an x–y graph, more difficult to interpret a 3-D graph, and virtually impossible to contemplate a 7-dimension, 7-axis coordinate system. Fortunately, computer software is not confused by higher dimensional analysis. Multiple subscripts can get confusing, so developing a structured approach to high-dimension data is critically important.

5.4   Summary of Vector and Matrix Rules

Modern computers have made vector and matrix mathematics straightforward—as long as the rules are followed—but performing matrix operations using software may require specific formatting (an exception is the software Matlab, which does matrix operations intuitively). As a "health systems engineer" you don't need to be able to do matrix operations, but you do need to understand what they are and how to interpret them in a book or article. There are a few operations, in particular, that should be understood.

1. Transposing a vector converts it from a row to a column or vice versa. Typically a vector, a, in a written equation is a <u>column vector by default</u>, so the transpose, a', is a row vector. In many textbooks, when an equation appears in a line of text, x is considered a row vector, so a column vector could be indicated by x'. This can be confusing, so be aware!
2. Two vectors can be multiplied two ways, determined by the order. Vector/matrix multiplication is always performed "row by column" (that is by going across the row of the first vector and down the column of the second). So remember the phrase "row by column." Multiplying a row vector <u>on the left</u> by a column vector <u>on the right</u> (for example (1×5) times (5×1) is the sum of all of the resulting paired multiples, a scalar not a vector result. This is known as the dot product $(\mathbf{x}{\cdot}\mathbf{y})$. This is noteworthy as a measure of statistical independence, because when the dot product is NOT equal to zero, the vectors are not orthogonal (perpendicular) and not independent. (Usually the opposite is also true, if the dot product is zero, the vectors are orthogonal—BUT NOT ALWAYS.) Another important example uses the dot product to determine a sum of squares. After centering a vector by subtracting its mean, multiplying it as a row (on the left) by itself as a

column (**xx'**) results in the sum of squared residuals. Excel can perform this using the = SUMPRODUCT function.
3. Multiplying with a column vector on the left and a row vector on the right (such as a (5×1) times a (1×4) produces a full (5×4) matrix. A matrix has dimension $R \times C$; a vector can be considered a matrix with one dimension equal to "1." An $R \times 1$ matrix is a column vector; a $1 \times C$ matrix is a row vector. Multiplying two matrices $(R1 \times C1) \times (R2 \times C2)$ always requires that the inside C1 and R2 are identical, and the dimension of the resulting matrix is $R1 \times C2$. So multiplying a column vector Rx1 (read R rows by 1 column) by a row vector $1 \times C$ (1 row by C columns) gives an $R \times C$ matrix as a result.
4. As previously stated, multiplying a centered row vector by the transpose (a column vector) produces a sum of squares. Multiplying a centered <u>matrix</u> (**X**) by the transpose of itself (**X'**) and dividing each resulting element by n results in the covariance matrix.

5.5   The Curse of Dimensionality and the Bias-Variance Trade-Off

The term "curse of dimensionality" introduces the dilemma of size. Large size is often considered beneficial in statistics, as it provides more accurate estimates of the parameters of a set of numbers (reduced bias). This can also be true for the number of variables in a dataset, for the same reason. However, as the number of variables in a dataset increases, the sum of squared residuals (and thus the variance) increases progressively. When building a model from a dataset with a large number of included variables (columns), we would like to develop an equation that accurately represents the outcomes of the dataset itself and that also predicts the result for a new set of inputs. But all models contain "error" -random error due to variability and chance, systematic error due to biased measurements. Testing the model against the data that were used to construct it gives "training error" (internal error). Testing it against a new set of data gives "generalization error" (external error). It is not uncommon in the medical literature for a model to be "validated" using the same data that were used to create it. But this only tests training error and says nothing about whether the model can be of any usefulness when applied to a new set of data (generalization error). Each time we introduce an additional variable into a model, two things happen: we improve the measurement of the "average" but then, after initially improving variance, the variance begins to increase. This is called **the curse of dimensionality** [1]. Our goal is to identify just the right number of variables that minimizes the internal error while not increasing the generalization error.

Start building a model, using only one of the input columns (the one most highly correlated with the outcome column from the combined correlation matrix). With only a **single** input variable, there will likely be a large difference between the <u>actual</u> outcome in the dataset and the <u>predicted</u> outcome. This is the "bias." If we next build a model with the best **two** input variables, the bias will still be large, but smaller than with only one. Each time an additional variable is added, the model appears to be

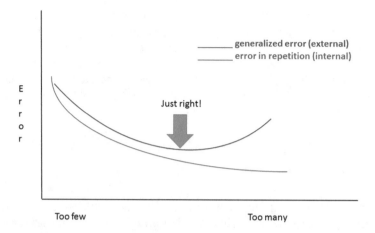

Fig. 5.1 Effect of the number of variables (model complexity) on the internal (training) error and the external (generalization) error. Too few input variables increases bias (difference between observed and expected), while too many increases variance. The "correct" number of input variables is much like the quote from Goldilocks—not too small, not too large, just right. It is tempting to want to include ALL of the variables, believing that this will produce the best model. Understanding the Goldilocks principle and the "curse of dimensionality" should result in an "optimal" model

better because the bias decreases further. Hence, increasing the number of variables in the model predicts the original data set better and better by reducing bias.

However, something different occurs when a model is applied to a NEW set of data. In applying each of these models, starting with one input variable, to a new set of data, the generalization error at first decreases as each variable is added but then the error increases, because the model is adding additional "unnecessary" data. This means that predictive ability improves up to a point and then decreases as the intrinsic variance of the model begins to increase (generalization error).

So if the model has too few input variables, it has high bias. If it has too many input variables, it has high variance. This is like the Goldilocks phenomenon—not too small, not too large, just right (Fig. 5.1). A key ability in analytics is to overlook the temptation to build BIG models, using ALL of the input variables under the false sense that it is somehow better. There is a BEST size for any model—fewer or more input variables than the optimum will degrade the model. This is the curse of dimensionality. But fortunately, there are ways to "estimate" these errors and "right-size" the number of input variables.

5.6   Factors That Degrade Models

5.6.1   Cause and Effect

There is a difference between an association and a cause-and-effect relationship [2–4]. Demonstrating a correlation could represent only an association or it could actually indicate a cause-and-effect relationship, but unfortunately it is not possible to determine which in a retrospective analysis. Actual cause and effect can ONLY be <u>definitively</u> established in a designed, prospective randomized analysis in which all of the other possible causes have been "controlled." Retrospective data analysis is based on inference (inductive reasoning) and can <u>establish</u> an association or relationship but only <u>SUGGEST</u> the possibility of cause and effect. It is tempting to infer that a strong correlation indicates cause and effect, but this is often incorrect, due to Simpson's Paradox [1] (see below).

5.6.2   Collinearity

Since so many things in the human body and within the health care environment are "connected" to each other, it should not be a surprise that many of the measurements we make and the resulting data we use consist of things that vary together in consistent ways. Some are obvious, such as body weight and BMI, which typically have about a 95% correlation. But many others are not obvious at all—because of Simpson's paradox. Formally, Simpson's paradox is said to occur when a difference in smaller groups disappears when the groups are combined, but a variation on that explanation is more helpful—Simpson's paradox is due to the false attribution of cause and effect when in fact both measures are the result of something else, unmeasured. A textbook example is the relationship between arm length and reading ability, which disappears when age is fixed—an 18-year-old has longer arms and better reading ability than a 4-year-old, but that is hardly cause and effect. Rather, each is the consequence of age related development. Many of the measurements commonly used in medical diagnosis and treatment are actually surrogate measures of more fundamental factors NOT included in the dataset—serum cholesterol level is actually a surrogate measure for a number of complex biochemical and genetic factors, and not actually "causal." Hemoglobin A1C is a surrogate measure for the severity of diabetes and the effectiveness of treatment, so a drug that only lowered the HbA1C might not be expected to lessen diabetic neuropathy. The first step in understanding a set of data must be to determine how extensive and how strong the correlations among variables are, using a correlation matrix. As previously described, the correlation matrix is square and symmetrical with "1s" on the diagonal. Each off-diagonal value is the correlation coefficient for the indicated pair of variables, ranging from −1 to +1. When the correlation coefficient is squared, it is known as **R-squared** or the **coefficient of determination,** which estimates the percentage of the total variance that is explained by that variable (as opposed to random noise). As rough rules of thumb, use <0.1 = minimal correlation, >0.4 = some, and >0.9 = strong. When additional variables are added to a model, by definition the unadjusted variance increases. As we will see when we build models, a multi-variable R-squared can be further adjusted for the spurious impact of just adding another variable (R^2_{adj}), and can be further manipulated to determine the variance inflation factor (VIF). A VIF>5 is suggestive and >10 indicative of collinearity which can significantly impact the interpretive ability of a model. The simplest way to think about collinearity is that correlated variables contribute more than their proper contribution to a model (including both BMI and weight is analogous to including either one twice!). There are many ways to address multicollinearity when it is identified: do nothing and explain the limitations of the model, eliminate highly collinear variables, or create new input variables that are mathematically uncorrelated (ridge regression, lasso regression, and principal component regression). Remember that correlation of input variables implies collinearity and suggests a possible Simpson's paradox.

5.6.3 Proximity, Distances, and Similarities

Most analytical methods are based on some measure of proximity (closeness), which can be a quantitative **distance** or a qualitative/semiquantitative **similarity** [1]. We are accustomed to measures of distance in our real, three-dimensional world (**Euclidean distance**) and to similarities that are perceived with our senses (**concordance**). Analytical proximity often occurs in a multidimensional space or using different similarities.

Many measures of similarity are based on percent agreement (e.g., **simple matching coefficient**, **Jaccard coefficient**) but others are less obvious (density, nearest neighbors). Similarly, there are other measures of distance (**Manhattan distance**, known as L1, best thought of as how one would drive from one point to another in a major city). In fact, there is a whole family of distances based on increasing exponential powers (L1-Manhattan; L2-Euclidean; L∞–Supremum) in the relationship known as the generalized Minkowski distance:

$$d(x,y) = \left(\Sigma \left(|x_i - y_i|^r \right) \right)^{1/r}$$

where $d(x, y)$, the distance between x and y, is the rth root of the sum of the absolute difference raised to the rth power. Inspection will confirm that when $r=1$, it is the Manhattan; $r=2$, Euclidean, etc. Each of these corresponds to a difference between points, vectors, or arrays in a dimensional space. Often we are interested in how far a point is from a distribution of values, for example in identifying **outlier** values.

The **Mahalanobis distance** is the measure of the squared difference between a single point in space and a set of multidimensional points with a **centroid** and a covariance matrix defining the distribution of the comparison points. It can be determined in Minitab (Stat:Multivariate:PrincipalComponents:Graphs:Outlier) and "R" (mahalanobis()). It can be thought of as a z-score using a multidimensional hypotenuse—the number of multidimensional standardized units—and is thus useful in identifying potential outliers or in estimating an adjusted multidimensional "distance" metric.

5.6.4 Sample Size: What Is Small

Increasing sample size is a generally understood concept in statistics, yet aggregated and retrospective data come with a predetermined size. Understanding the importance of the actual sample size is just as important as increasing sample size in a prospective study. Conceptually, the question "what is small" is probably more useful than "what is large," because bias noticeably increases when $n < 30$ [5]. Examination of the t-table reaffirms that t-values level off at $n > 30$. Therefore this number is widely accepted as the cutoff between "small" and "not-small." Even when the total sample is very large, if a subset is less than 30, it must be considered "small" and dealt with (analysis as well as interpretation) accordingly. Another aspect of size consideration is in examining distributions. Both the binomial distribution (yes/no) and the Poisson distribution (counts) are known to approach the normal distribution with large sample size. Again, consideration of small is more useful—either distribution will be VERY non-normal when $n < 30$ and somewhat non-normal for $30 < n < 100$.

5.6.5 Understanding Hypothesis Testing

Many students seem to have difficulty understanding exactly what is happening during hypothesis testing. **Hypothesis testing** is the critical thought process in the **scientific method**:

- Identify what you "hope" to find.
- Turn it around into a null hypothesis (H_0:).
- Test the null hypothesis and either accept or reject it.
- If reject the null, then accept the alternative hypothesis.
- Otherwise accept the null (H_1).

There are two sites for error: first, in rejecting the null hypothesis; second, in NOT rejecting the null hypothesis. In both cases, a p-value is involved: α-alpha, ($P(R|T)$, the conditional probability of rejecting the null given that the null is true), and β-beta, ($P(A|F)$, the conditional probability of accepting the null given that the null is false). In both cases, the p-value is a BELIEF STATEMENT of how willing one is to be wrong (and NOT a proof of concept statement!) If I reject the null, with a defined $p < 0.05$, I am saying that by rejecting the null I am accepting that I could be wrong up to 5 % of the time. Although 5 % is the typical default, is that number appropriate for the risk I'm willing to take? In cancer research should I be more liberal? In designing a space shuttle, should I be more stringent?

Not well understood by many investigators, β (the likelihood of being wrong if you accept the null hypothesis) is typically much larger, in the order of 10–30 %, which means that if I ACCEPT the null of no difference, I am willing to be wrong that often. Compare this to the weather report: 5 % chance of rain means that on days similar to this, 1 in 20 had rain—will it rain? In analysis and modeling, it is critically important to avoid the temptation to say that the p-value indicates importance, usefulness, or value, none of which is correct. Also critically important is the realization that the alternate hypothesis was never actually tested—it was simply what we set up in the beginning as the alternate. Again using weather, if the choice of hypotheses is rain or no rain, what about snow?

5.6.6 Applying Probability and Statistics

Most physicians view probability and statistics as either an undergraduate course they would like not to remember or a necessary component of publishing a manuscript. It is perhaps preferable to think of it as a broadly based approach to understanding uncertainty—uncertainty in medicine, in research, and in life. A bit of background may be helpful.

The concept of probability is attributed to Blaise Pascal (1623–1662) [6], French philosopher-mathematician remembered for Pascal's triangle, who wanted to improve his results at gambling. He proposed what we now call the binomial theorem. Probability continued to develop over the next 200 years, still focused almost exclusively on gambling. Carl Friedrich Gauss (1777–1855), a German professor of mathematics, applied the recently discovered "calculus" to generalize the binomial to a continuous distribution, as an applied mathematics exercise. Over the ensuing years, many natural phenomena were noted to follow this "Gaussian" distribution, and so it acquired the name "normal." Normal at that time was heavily related to agriculture, and plant growth behavior largely conforms to the binomial. As the agricultural revolution matured and evolved into the technical revolution, it continued to be about farming. George Snedecor (1881–1974) in the USA and Ronald Fisher (1899–1962) in England independently developed programs which applied probability theory directly to farming in order to inform farmers of the benefits and safety of investing their hard-earned resources into newly developed agriculture concepts and technology, naming the new discipline "statistics" [7]. Early statistics were exclusively based on a world that followed the "normal" (Gaussian) distribution, but soon it became apparent that many things did NOT conform to a bell-shaped curve. Two approaches were introduced to address this "non-normality," non-parametric statistics and statistical transformations. The former was a likelihood-based approach that made no assumption of an underlying distribution, and the latter found ways to transform data so as to conform to the normal distribution. Arguments would ensue over the next three-quarters of a century about normality and statistics. In the 1990s, a concept known as **conditional probability** reemerged on the statistics scene [8]. Originally described by Thomas Bayes (1701–1761), a British Protestant minister, and advanced by Pierre-Simon Laplace (1749–1827), Bayes' theorem was actively resisted by the scientific community and survived "clandestinely" through 200 years. It achieved great although unheralded success during World War II in the emerging field of Operations Research, which revolutionized war planning and saved the British from the German blitzkrieg and submarine wolfpacks as well as provided sufficient and timely materiel, provisions, and resources for two separate theaters of war, half a world apart [9]. Rediscovered and popularized in the 1990s, Bayesian logic and analysis have been principal drivers in advancing the field of applied statistics, including in medicine. Described briefly earlier, Bayes' theorem allows back-and-forth movement between a "prior probability" of a disease ($P(D)$) and a modified "posterior probability," $P(D|+)$—the likelihood of the disease given a positive test:

$$P(D\,|\,+) = P(+\,|\,D) \times \frac{P(D)}{P(+)}$$

Everything in medicine is stochastic, subject to uncertainty and error. Every number should be thought of as a distribution of possible numbers with a central tendency and a likely range.

References

1. Tan PNSM, Kumar V. Introduction to data mining. Boston: Pearson-Addison Wesley; 2006. p. 22–36.
2. Lucas RM, McMichael AJ. Association or causation: evaluating links between "environment and disease". Bull World Health Organ. 2005;83(10):792–5.
3. Matt V, Matthew H. The retrospective chart review: important methodological considerations. J Educ Eval Health Prof. 2013;10:12.
4. Morgan SL, Winship C. Counterfactuals and causal inference: methods and principles for social research, vol. xiii. New York: Cambridge University Press; 2007. 319 p.
5. Hand DJ. The improbability principle: why coincidences, miracles, and rare events happen every day. 1st ed. New York: Scientific American; 2014.
6. Franklin J. The science of conjecture: evidence and probability before Pascal, vol. xiii. Baltimore: Johns Hopkins University Press; 2001. 497 p.
7. Stigler SM. Statistics on the table: the history of statistical concepts and methods, vol. ix. Cambridge, MA: Harvard University Press; 1999. 488 p.
8. McGrayne SB. The theory that would not die: how Bayes' rule cracked the enigma code, hunted down Russian submarines, & emerged triumphant from two centuries of controversy, vol. xiii. New Haven, CT: Yale University Press; 2011. 320 p.
9. Budiansky S. Blackett's war. 1st ed. New York: Alfred A. Knopf; 2013. 306 p.

Part III
Techniques in Analysis

Chapter 6
Analysis by Modeling Data

Scenario

Dr. Joyce Smith is a successful neonatologist. She is approached by the nurse manager of the neonatal ICU because the method they are using to store mothers' breast milk, brought in small vials in cardboard boxes, isn't working. Often the vials sit in the refrigerator until they passed the expiration date. Sometimes milk is given to the wrong infant. Commonly, some babies have more milk available than they can use and others have none. Joyce has an idea and meets with the produce manager at the local grocery store, part of a large national chain. She learns that they have computer systems that track every single piece of produce, identify the expected needs by week of the year, update based on holidays, track seasonal changes, and maintain a "just-in-time" inventory that avoids spoilage but also shortages. They also use a tracking system that scans in every package of produce, automatically producing labels that are scanned at checkout. Experts regularly update predictive computer models of usage and trends (**database; marketbaskettime series; predictive regression models**).

6.1 Preparing to Build Models

After completing the initial analysis of the structure and composition of the data, formal analysis typically requires creation of a **model** [1]. A model is a replica or representation, typically simpler than the reality. A doll house is a model of a real house. Nevertheless it is tempting to believe that, like Geppetto's puppet Pinocchio, the model can become real. George Box, one of the premiere statisticians of the late twentieth century, reminded us that "All models are wrong, but some models are useful [1]." By their nature, data are "messy," but models are "neat." Because of

© Springer International Publishing Switzerland 2016
P.J. Fabri, *Measurement and Analysis in Transforming Healthcare Delivery*,
DOI 10.1007/978-3-319-40812-5_6

the neatness and simplicity of models, it is a common mistake to replace the reality with the model and its components, ignoring the messiness and uncertainty. It is important always to be reminded that a model is just a model.

Uncertainty is an unavoidable reality of data analysis. Because the data are physically in the computer, it is easy to forget that the data are only one of an infinite variety of datasets that COULD have been collected. The current dataset is a SAMPLE from a very large POPULATION. The model must be able to generalize to the larger population to be meaningful and useful. Progressively more detailed modeling, triggered by the belief that the data ARE the reality, can easily result in models that look better and better while actually being less able to be generalized— overfitting. In order to avoid two important errors, mistaking the model for reality and overfitting the model, it is important to understand the role of hypothesis testing and validation in modeling.

6.1.1   The Model in Light of the Hypothesis [2]

The **hypothesis** is the construct against which statistical tests are framed. In a prospective study, the hypothesis is established in advance. In a retrospective analysis, the hypothesis is surmised from looking at the data. In a prospective analysis, all of the covariates have been fixed, so that the experiment focuses on the question at hand, allowing a deductive conclusion—if the null hypothesis is rejected, the predefined alternate must be the answer. In a retrospective analysis, where the variables are only a "convenience sample" of all of the possible variables and the dataset just another "convenience sample" of all the possible subjects, only an inductive answer is possible. In other words, in a prospective study, the null and alternate hypotheses are clear; in a retrospective model if the null hypothesis is rejected, the alternate can only be "it isn't the null hypothesis," and therefore of all the possible alternatives this seems most likely. For this reason, a retrospective analysis CANNOT establish definitely a cause-and-effect relationship, only a likelihood. Increasing rigor in selecting and applying analytic methods can increase the likelihood, but not establish certainty. Consider the example of looking for a new house. Your realtor has assembled a detailed and accurate report describing year of construction, all of the room dimensions plus ceiling heights, number of rooms, total square feet, number of bedrooms and bathrooms, number of fireplaces, and date of kitchen remodeling (in other words, a thorough dataset). If someone then tried to build that house from scratch (or a model of it) how many different ways could that house be built? If the realtor had collected a modestly different set of data, would the model be the same?

6.1.2   Planning to Validate a Model

Validation is the use of additional methods to affirm that the model "works" [3, 4]. Once again, it is tempting to accept that, because a model accurately predicts the data that created it, the model has been validated. But realizing that the data that made it were "sampled" (a defined subset of patients, this hospital versus that hospital, this insurance company, this healthcare system, etc.) only affirms that these data are not necessarily the same as other data that COULD have been obtained. For this reason, an objective method that establishes the generalizability of the model is necessary. Most analysts still hold that the ideal method to validate a model, given a sufficient sample size, is to apply it to a new, unrelated set of data that was never used in model development. In a perfect world, this would be a new set of data from an entirely different sampling. More realistically, this is a subset of the original dataset that is set aside specifically for this purpose in advance. Many investigators will divide a dataset into three subsets, a training set (to build the models), a test set (to select the best from among the models), and a validation set (to affirm that the chosen model works). 80:10:10 is a reasonable approach IF 10% of the total sample is "not small," but other ratios are also reasonable. The training set is used repeatedly to build a number of different models, each of which addresses some limitation of the assumptions. The test set is used repeatedly to measure the accuracy of the models. The validation set is not touched until all of this is completed—only then is it "taken out of the safe" and used for final validation that the model works. But often the total dataset is too small to allow partitioning. To address this, alternate methods have been developed: cross-validation, jackknife analysis, and bootstrapping.

6.1.3   Validation Methods When Partitioning Isn't Feasible

When the total number of records is small, requiring that all be used in building the model, alternative methods of validation must be used. Each of these creates new samples from the original dataset, allowing training sets and test sets to be constructed several times using the same modeling approach. This allows an assessment of the repeatability of a model. It assumes that the original dataset is "fair" and "unbiased" and that it truly represents the problem being addressed. If this assumption is made, there are three approaches to "internal" validation, cross-validation, jackknife, and bootstrap.

Cross-validation [5]: Cross-validation is probably the most "acceptable" method to validate a model when the sample size is limited. Cross-validation consists of dividing the dataset randomly into a fixed number of subsets, typically ten (although five may be more realistic with a small sample). One at a time, each of these subsets is defined as the "test" set, and the other 90% is used to create a model. Each of the ten uses a slightly different set of training data, and each of the test sets is "new" to that model. The variability of the models is assessed by a modification of the Chi-squared distribution known as the Hosmer-Lemeshow test. If the variability is "small," the model is considered valid. Note, however, that all of the data originated from the same sample, and most of the training sets are repetitions.

Jackknife analysis [5], also known as leave-one-out, would appear to be the "ultimate" cross-validation, selecting one at a time each of the data points as the "test" and building n models, each with $n-1$ training data points. Many authors believe that this approach is susceptible to greater bias, since the n models are very highly correlated (reference). Nevertheless many software packages provide this as an additional validation method for smaller datasets.

Bootstrap analysis [5] is a clever compromise which, unlike cross-validation that only really says "yes" or "no" to the variability of the ten models, provides an actual distribution of validation outcomes. To perform bootstrapping, a random sample of size "n" is taken WITH REPLACEMENT, which means that some data points will be sampled more than once. These "n" data points are used to create a model, which is then tested against the data points that were not selected. This is repeated, over and over, a specified number of times (for example a 1000-fold bootstrap). The parameters of each of these outcomes can be visualized as a distribution function that characterizes that model, since, although the applied data vary, the model stays the same. A distinct advantage of bootstrapping is that the probability of a data point being included stays constant because of replacement. A theoretical limitation is that data points are repeated in the models, although it is random. Bootstrapping requires a fast computer and the attendant software, whereas cross-validation could theoretically be done by hand.

Ideally, a separate test set and validation set should be set aside before model-building. When this is unrealistic because of a small number of records, the "internal" validation methods provide an assessment of repeatability but not true "generalizability." Whichever method is selected, ALL MODELS should be validated, with a formal measurement of intrinsic bias (within the training set) and extrinsic variance (in a "new" dataset). This validation process defines a model's usefulness and quantifies the bias-variance trade-off.

Because all modeling efforts make initial assumptions, which are often only partially met, alternative modeling approaches should also be used. If several different approaches provide essentially the same answer, modeling is likely to be valid. If different approaches yield very different answers, the accuracy of modeling should be questioned. When multiple methods have been used, the simplest method to assess "the best" is to measure the mean squared error (MSE) from the residuals as the model is applied to the test data. More elegant (but complicated) methods exist, based on an estimation of the log-likelihood loss function [5]. The two most often applied are the Akaike Information Criterion (AIC) and the Bayesian Information Criterion (BIC). They are very closely related, and the AIC seems to be slightly preferable. The software is typically programmed to do one or the other, so that the analyst should be conceptually familiar with both and comfortable with either. As an oversimplified explanation, the AIC tends to select slightly more complex models, while the BIC tends to favor slightly simpler models. To the individual analyst, the choice of metric is less important than having a metric and using it consistently. In the final analysis, a model is useful if it works, and the best choice of models is the one that works best. Using only one modeling approach and accepting it as "good" provides no assessment of how good! After a model has been created in R, the AIC can be determined for it (and other trial models) by clicking on it in the **Rcmdr** Models menu.

6.1.4   Planning to Combine Models: The Ensemble Approach

The term **ensemble** means "a group of items viewed as a whole rather than individually," or "a group or unit of complementary parts that contribute to a single effect." In analytics, creating an ensemble means combining together a variety of different approaches in order to produce a more useful aggregate model that benefits from the strengths of each of the components. A useful example is in the approach of the National Weather Service in forecasting tropical weather (Fig. 6.1). During hurricane season (June 1 to November 30), tropical weather forecasts are created independently by numerous meteorological agencies around the world. The National Hurricane Center (a division of the NOAA) issues a comprehensive analysis and forecast every 6 h (Global Ensemble Forecast System-GEFS). The NHC forecast includes many individual models but also includes an ensemble model that combines together a set of 22 different models, with 6 heavily weighted major models. The ensemble model is then iteratively applied to a dataset a large number of times, each time just barely "tweaking" the data to see how much the outcome predictions vary with small amounts of uncertainty (spaghetti models). They then look back, days later, to see how well the ensemble model matched the real storm, using the analysis of how each component in the model performed to adjust the weights of the models for the next storm. Why do they do this? To quote the NHC, "Although the deterministic approach has served us well, it is STEEPED IN ERROR, and will NEVER produce a perfect model" (http://www.hpc.ncep.noaa.gov/ensembletraining/). Note that the NHC makes no attempt to identify which of the input variables CAUSE the behavior of the storm! Their goal is not to establish causation but to produce a model that works.

In analyzing healthcare data, it is equally reasonable to combine different models (see for example the different approaches to regression) into an ensemble model to take advantage of the strengths of each. Several specific approaches to ensembles

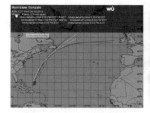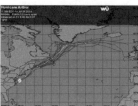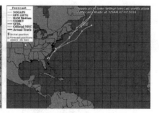

Fig. 6.1   An excellent example of "modeling," familiar to most, is demonstrated in hurricane prediction by the National Weather Service. (**a**) Shows predictive models from six different expert meteorological organizations, modeled from essentially the same dataset, showing how different models can originate from the same data. In some hurricanes, the difference in the models can be dramatic. (**b**) Shows the "consensus model" in *white*, which is the weighted aggregate of all of the individual models. The *pink* "spaghetti" demonstrates sensitivity analysis, achieved by running the consensus model over and over, each time with very slight changes in the input data to determine how robust the model is to small errors in the data. (**c**) The NHC routinely "validates" the models AFTER the storm to see how well the consensus model performed (*solid black line*)

have been developed. **Bagging** [5] involves **b**ootstrap **agg**regating to produce an "averaged" model; **boosting** [5] uses the data points that were hardest to fit (weak learners) to produce a model tailored to address the "difficulties"; **stacking** [5] (stacked generalization) applies machine learning to a set of models built with machine learning and "stacks" them together.

6.2   Building Models: Supervised and Unsupervised Machine Learning

6.2.1   Types of Models

Using computers to create analytical models is "machine learning." If an outcome variable is included, it is called "supervised" and if not, "unsupervised." Machine learning, then, whether supervised or unsupervised, is building models. Supervised learning has outcomes to evaluate accuracy, while unsupervised learning can only generate "concepts." Supervised learning produces "predictive" models, while unsupervised learning can only generate "understanding" models. Regression methods (continuous outcome data) and classification methods (categorical outcomes, usually binary), being supervised, generate predictive models. Association analysis (qualitative data) and cluster analysis (quantitative data without outcome) improve conceptual understanding.

Visualizing and quantifying changes over time produce a **time series** [6], while modeling "failure" (failure of a machine, death of a patient, etc.) over time uses **hazard functions** and **survival curves** [7].

6.2.2   The Problem of Unbalanced Datasets

It is not uncommon that important subgroups in a dataset are not represented equally or are subject to some other lack of balance such as patient selection or referral bias (e.g., academic quaternary hospital), hospital non-representativeness (e.g., national reputation for a particular operation or procedure or atypical patient populations such as veterans, immigrants, religious groups), etc. Such lack of balance can affect both the generalizablility of the outcomes as well as the structure of the models themselves. In a retrospective analysis or non-randomized "observational" prospective analysis, inferring a causal relationship requires structured selection of subgroups in order to create the "best" model, in essence "mimicking" a PRCT with groups that have been adjusted to approximate balance. Commonly, for example, patients experiencing a complication are numerically much less frequent than patients who don't, have very different patterns of comorbidity, are more likely to have been referred, etc. In other words, they are probably not truly comparable. So they need to be "restructured" to make them as comparable as possible, adjusting for underlying differences in groups.

6.2.2.1 Selecting a Random Subgroup of Reference Subjects

If there are unequal numbers in subgroups, the "study" group (e.g., "died," "was readmitted," or "had a complication") is usually small compared to the "reference" group, but there is otherwise no evidence of "bias." If there is no reason to believe that the qualitative aspects of the subjects are different, a "fair" method of balancing the model is to randomly select from the reference group on a 1:1 or 2:1 basis. While not using all of the data may seem to limit an analysis, in fact it usually produces a more valid and representative model by "approximating" the balance of a PRCT. A more "balanced" analysis is now possible.

6.2.2.2 Adjusting "Biased" Subgroups

Most healthcare datasets DO contain serious biases, such as fundamental differences in socioeconomic factors, multicollinear variables, or lack of important explanatory data. None of these can be "corrected" by selecting a random, matching-size reference group. Although random error decreases with larger sample size, nonrandom error due to bias stays the same, so that the proportion of error due to bias actually increases. This increase in bias requires an active approach to assure that the groups being analyzed are comparable enough to be able to isolate real differences.

Two useful approaches to dealing with these nonrandom errors are **propensity scores** and **instrumental variables** [8]. Both methods are designed to improve the comparability of groups and minimize balance and bias problems, but in differing ways. In both cases, preliminary analysis characterizes subjects in a way that creates comparability and minimizes treatment bias. An important difference between them is that propensity scores are determined FROM THE DATA while instrumental variables are selected by INFERENCE. A **propensity score** assumes that all of the necessary factors to identify both treatment and outcome are represented in the data. The propensity score is then calculated AFTER setting aside a small number of factors considered potentially causative, creating a predictive model using all other "important" covariates (for example, age, gender, pay-status). This model-based propensity score can then be used, for example, to match each patient who required readmission to the hospital after a particular procedure with a non-readmission patient WITH THE SAME PROPENSITY SCORE. The subsequent model, then, will have more balanced groups and will focus only on the factors believed to be causally important. Note again that use of propensity scores assumes that "all the facts" are known and in the dataset. This is problematic when using a retrospective dataset, as many important variables are probably not captured.

Instrumental variables assume that important input variables are missing, sample selection is biased, or both. An instrumental variable is some specific input that is thought to provide a deeper level of understanding of the subjects that is not included in the dataset, yet does not itself influence the outcome. It is notably difficult to identify good instrumental variables, but when found they contribute substantially to model-building by comparing "oranges with oranges" instead of "apples." Instrumental variables must first make sense—they are reasonable and relevant. Zip Code may affect which hospital a patient is taken to by paramedics but does not INDEPENDENTLY affect mortality except by its influence on treatment. Once established as relevant and uncorrelated with outcome, an instrumental variable can be used in a **two-step regression** progress, the first step establishing the relationship between the instrumental variable and the treatment followed by the model-building regression utilizing the instrumental variable as an input predictor.

References

1. Box GEP. Robustness in the strategy of scientific model building. In: Launer RL, Wilkinson GN, editors. Robustness in statistics. New York: Academic; 1979.
2. Matt V, Matthew H. The retrospective chart review: important methodological considerations. J Educ Eval Health Prof. 2013;10:12.
3. Tan PN, Steinbach M, Kumar V. Introduction to Data Mining. Boston: Pearson-Addison Wesley; 2006. 769 p.
4. Altman DG, Royston P. What do we mean by validating a prognostic model? Stat Med. 2000;19(4):453–73.
5. Hastie T, Friedman JH, Tibshirani R. The elements of statistical learning: data mining, inference, and prediction. 2, corrected 7 printing edth ed. New York: Springer; 2009.
6. Shumway RH, Stoffer DS. Time series analysis and its applications: with R examples. New York: Springer Science & Business Media; 2010.
7. Bailar JC, Hoaglin DC. Medical uses of statistics. New York: Wiley; 2012.
8. Winship CW, Morgan SL. The estimation of causal effects from observational data. Annu Rev Sociol. 1999;25(1):659–706.

Chapter 7
Principles of Supervised Learning

Scenario

Dr. Ron Shepherd is the chief of colorectal surgery at a major academic medical center. He has been informed that the readmission rate for elective colorectal surgery is twice the national average. He convenes the division members to analyze the data in their database to see if they can identify potential contributing factors. Their review of the literature is not particularly helpful because no two published articles on colorectal readmissions provide even similar answers. Ron enlists the help of a systems engineer to help them determine the factors associated with readmission as well as a likelihood analysis of which of the factors might actually be part of the cause. Because of the high correlation among the variables in the dataset, they are going to use ridge classification and partial least square discriminant analysis. They are going to use ten-folk cross-validation and a final validation set to verify that the model can be generalized.

7.1 An Introduction to Supervised Machine Learning: Regression and Classification

Most physicians are at least vaguely familiar with the concepts of regression and logistic regression from reading the medical literature. These are the traditional workhorses of **supervised machine learning**. The ready availability of powerful computers allowed the development of newer approaches to the activities of regression and classification, which attempt to address the problems of meeting the assumptions inherent in the traditional approaches. Regression and classification models are similar in their approach, using a training set of data, validating the

© Springer International Publishing Switzerland 2016
P.J. Fabri, *Measurement and Analysis in Transforming Healthcare Delivery*,
DOI 10.1007/978-3-319-40812-5_7

model, and then applying that model to new data for the purposes of predicting. The model can be thought of as

$$\text{Inputs} \xrightarrow[\text{Transformation}]{} \text{Outputs}$$

The inputs are the set of input predictor variables "X," and the outputs are the predicted result after the application of the model "Y." The structure of the inputs is similar in both regression and classification, but the outputs are different-continuous and unconstrained in regression versus categorical and constrained in classification. Constraining the outcome in classification requires a different transformation approach than used in regression.

Building a model can be thought of as three separate components: evaluating and modifying the distributions, the format, and the weightings of the **inputs**; evaluating and modifying the distribution of the **output**; and applying one of the three approaches to create the connecting, **transformation** relationship—minimizing the SSR (least squares), maximizing the likelihood (MLE), or maximizing the constraining hyperplane (support vector machines) (Table 7.1). Managing the inputs includes defining the distributions, transforming the variables, and creating new forms of the variables to address multicollinearity, non-normality, non-additivity, etc. Managing training regression outputs, which are numbers (continuous variables), is generally limited to transforming the observed **y** output in the dataset to make it "normal," and the subsequent predicted $\hat{y}$ outputs are also "numbers." (Note: Although it is possible to use multiple outcome variables using multivariate regression, interpreting the result is challenging and often questionable. Multivariate regression is often a separate graduate course! Accordingly, we will limit our focus to a single-outcome variable, which is typical in the medical literature.) The observed training classification output g, however, most often a discrete, binary (lived/died, readmitted/not readmitted), is converted to probabilities and constrained to a scale of 0/1 to produce the predicted outputs $\hat{g}$. Output predicted values are similarly constrained along the continuum from 0 to 1, giving a decimal fraction which is rounded up or down to obtain the constrained values (0,1). The connecting transformation can also include modifying the input AND creating the equation simultaneously (e.g., ridge regression in essence creates new independent variables at the same time as deriving the predictive equation) OR sequentially (principal component regression first creates new, independent input variables, then builds the equation).

Table 7.1 Common methods used in analysis

Least squares	• Minimizes sum of squared residuals mathematically • Used extensively in regression
Maximum likelihood estimation	• Optimizes the parameters/coefficients by maximizing the "fit" to normal • Used occasionally in regression, frequently in classification and clustering
Optimizing separating hyperplane	• Identifies "zone" (maximum between classes or minimum around points) • Support vector machines for classification or regression

In regression, all analytical methods attempt to find a line which best "fits" or represents the set of multidimensional data. If it is a straight line, linear regression; if not straight, nonlinear, which requires an additional mathematical transform or a nonparametric method. When applied, these methods WILL ALWAYS find a line, whether meaningful or not, but the diagnostics are essential to determine if the line is actually worth finding. Most regression methods minimize the sum of squared residuals to find the line, some use maximizing the likelihood estimate, and support vector regression finds the axis of the minimal confining regular polyhedral figure which contains (creates a regular structure around) the data. Some measure of amount of error is used to accomplish the interpretation of "how good," often analysis of variance (ANOVA).

In classification, all analytical methods attempt to find a line that separates the data into distinct "regions," typically above or below a "line," "plane," or "hyperplane" in multidimensional space. Most classification methods maximize a likelihood function, which essentially creates probabilities for each of the data points to belong to each of the groups. Some methods apply Bayes' theorem to estimate the probabilities (e.g., discriminant analysis), while others use iterative optimization to maximize likelihood in a variation of linear regression (e.g., logistic regression), rounding the decimal fraction up or down to determine which class. (Keep in mind that this could mean different classes for 0.499 and 0.501, essentially a coin toss but these data points would be assigned to 0 and 1.)

The application of the model to the original training data produces predicted values Y-hat (regression) or G-hat (classification), allowing residuals or differences to be assessed and evaluated. Applying the model to a separate subset of data validates the model. Keeping in mind that a model is only a model, the appropriateness of applying the model to a new set of data always requires the assumption that NOTHING HAS CHANGED along the way! Even then, however, models can be wrong.

7.2   Setting the Stage for Regression: An Example

The Accountable Care Act has introduced a new level of accountability in healthcare, which will require increased attentiveness to measuring and predicting a wide variety of quantitative outcomes. Hospitals will need to be able to predict length of stay and cost of treatment for specific conditions and understand the importance of associated factors. Some of these factors may actually be causal, while many of the variables will only be "coming along for the ride." Efforts to influence or change these "associated" factors, no matter how well planned, will unlikely alter the outcome, whereas programs that address true causative factors are more likely to effect substantive change. Solving these issues is the domain of regression models. Since a model is only a model, multiple modeling approaches should be conducted and compared to see which works best, keeping in mind that "causation" is unlikely to be achievable.

7.2.1   Principles of Regression

(For those interested, a comprehensive presentation of the principles of regression can be found in Kutner et al. [1].) Regression is defined as a measure of the relation between the mean value of one variable (output) and the corresponding values of other variables (inputs). In other words, it "explains" an outcome variable in terms of a set of inputs. Traditional regression methods assume that the only "uncertainty" is in the output, and the inputs are known without error. (This is called a fixed effect model, as opposed to a random effect model which includes uncertainty in the inputs but is much more complicated. Although probably appropriate much of the time, random effect models are uncommon!) Since the outcome variable in regression is traditionally referred to as "y," that means all of the error is assumed to be in the "y" direction (up or down). Regression, then, determines the equation of the "best-fit" straight line, through the x–y data points by minimizing the difference between the predicted y-value (y-hat or $\hat{y}$) at each level of "x" and the actual y value. Several approaches are available to "fit" the best-fit model to a set of data: by minimizing residuals, by maximizing likelihood, or by creating a support vector machine (Table 7.1). Mathematically, this is accomplished by optimizing the fit of a model to the training set by either **minimizing** the sum of squared residuals ($SSR = \Sigma (y - \hat{y})^2$) or **maximizing** the likelihood relative to a normal distribution. Minimizing the SSR can be accomplished two different ways: by calculation, setting the first derivative (rate of change) of the residuals to zero, or by optimization, **iteratively** determining the best parameters for a normal distribution of errors around the line using optimizing software like Solver. Details of the methodologies are readily available in standard references. While this is easiest to see in a two-dimension x–y plot, it can be generalized to any number of variables (dimensions) equivalently. Nonlinear curve fitting can also be performed but requires a suitable mathematical transformation of the data to fit a curve, followed by a similar process of optimization to determine the parameters.

7.2.2   Assumptions of Regression

Regression makes four primary assumptions (of a longer list of total assumptions as shown in Table 7.2) [2], and deviating from these assumptions degrades the accuracy of the model to a greater or lesser degree (regression assumptions:

Table 7.2 Assumptions of most models (of varying importance to validity)	
	• Normal distribution of variables
	• Normal distribution of residuals
	• Additivity of terms
	• Mathematical independence of variables
	• Non-collinearity of variables
	• Appropriate number of dimensions

normality of the residuals, errors are independent and not interactive, uniform distribution (homoscedasticity) and linearity/additivity of the terms). Sadly, red lights don't flash when these assumptions are violated, and many regression-based models are built with intrinsic flaws that limit the accuracy of the resulting conclusions. Although many statistical tests have been developed to identify these potential pitfalls, the easiest and best way to assess adherence to the assumptions is by creating a set of residual graphs [3]. Minitab creates a set of four graphs [4] (see Fig. 4.4) which visually characterize the residuals to determine if: the residuals adhere to a normal distribution in the **normal distribution plot**; the distribution of the data is markedly skewed in the **histogram**; the residuals are uniform across the range of input data in the **versus fit** plot; and the residuals vary as a function of time or sequence in the **versus order** plot. If all four graphs are "acceptable," normality of residuals and homoscedasticity are highly likely. Independence of the input variables is a separate issue, but is assessed by examining a correlation matrix.

7.2.3 Limitations of a Regression Model

Regression assumes that the real world can actually be modeled from a mathematical equation in a useful and predictive way. The fact that software can create a regression model does not mean that the model is appropriate or useful. The variables in the dataset may or may not be the most relevant to the actual outcome. Many other variables COULD have been measured/included in the database, some of which might have produced a much better model. Also, some of the "missing" variables might actually be causative. Additionally, the model might be applied outside its useful range. The model's mathematical equation is created (trained) from a set of input data that cover a specific range of inputs. It is tempting to extrapolate a predictive model outside of the range of the inputs. If there is a well-established scientific basis for a model (for example pressure = flow x resistance), the relationship MIGHT be expected to persist outside the range of the inputs, but if the modeling equation is empirically derived from the data, it is hazardous to extend predictions outside of the range of the data available to build the model. For example, is the effect of weight on developing coronary artery disease the same with a five-pound weight gain from 160 to 165 as from 400 to 405? Finally, keep in mind that even the venerable equations learned in physics class were inferred from data and often don't strictly hold!

Multiple regression depends similarly on the same assumptions. In addition, it is subject to dimensionality and causality. Thoughtful analysis will consider normality of residuals, uniformity of variance, linearity, additivity, independence, dimensionality, and cause/effect. It is the rare model that does not deviate in one or more ways from ideal, and this is the reason alternative methods have been developed in recent years. We will now consider additional approaches to regression.

7.2.4   Alternative Approaches to Regression

Although classical multiple regression has been the "standard approach" to modeling with a continuous outcome, more powerful modern computers have made it possible to create new modeling approaches that better address the limiting assumptions multiple regression presents. These methods typically "adapt" the input variables in order to address the inability to meet traditional assumptions (Table 7.3).

7.2.4.1   Methods to Select/Modify Input Variables

The typical database, containing a very large number of "fields," will contain unnecessary variables, highly correlated variables, and redundant variables which add no new information but complicate the model. Selecting the best variables (or more often removing the less desirable ones), based on information from a subject matter expert (SME) or from carefully examining a correlation matrix, is a good start. Rarely, however, will this remove a sufficient number of variables to improve dimensionality. After applying "logical" reasons to remove variables, it falls on the computer to decide. Three approaches are possible (Table 7.4): continued subset

Table 7.3 Methods for "adapting" input variables

• Mathematical weighting by
– History
– Formula
– Inverse of variance
• Penalty Function. Increases sum of squared residuals if coefficients increase (yin-yang)
– For example ridge regression and other penalized methods
– Variably shrinks <u>all</u> coefficients, eliminating none
• Forcing variables to zero
– A form of penalty function which actually eliminates some variables
– For example lasso (unlike ridge, it actually eliminates some)

Table 7.4 Methods for multiple regression

• Eliminating some variables
– Subject matter expert
– High correlation of variables (removes redundancy)
– Best subsets (tests all possible combinations)
– P-value on univariate regression (eliminates some variables)
• Shrinking contribution of variables (penalized regression)
– Ridge regression
– Lasso regression (forces some coefficients to zero, thus eliminating them)
– Least angle regression (a variant of lasso)
• Derived inputs (hybridized regression)
– Principle component regression (uses principle components as inputs)
– Partial least square regression (stepwise regression using residual variance)

narrowing, shrinking variables, and creating "better" variables from the existing ones [5]. A comprehensive discussion of these approaches can be found in Hastie et al. Only a brief summary is included here.

Subset narrowing—Analytical subset selection systematically works through all of the input variables based on their "contributions." It can be accomplished by stepwise addition (forward stepwise), stepwise deletion (backward stepwise), add one-subtract one (forward-backward stepwise), or best subsets (iteratively try every possible subset and select the best).

In forward stepwise regression, the variable with the "best" univariate result is entered first, then the second best, etc., until a stopping point has been reached (typically either an estimated probability cutoff or the lowest measure of accuracy such as mean square error or Akaike Information Criteria) or all of the original variables have been reintroduced. The latter accomplishes nothing except reordering the variables, but stopping sooner saves "the best" variables based on their performance WITHIN THIS DATASET. Its major concern is that which variable is entered first (and second, etc.) affects the order of entry of the remaining variables and thus changes the model. So if the "best" variable in THIS DATASET isn't actually the best variable (sampling error), the model will be adversely affected.

In backward stepwise regression, starting with all of the variables in the model, the "worst" variable is deleted, and so forth, until a stopping rule is reached. While this might seem to be the same as "forward," the risk of removing the "worst" versus the "second worst" is quite different than entering the "best" or the "second best," as it typically has no impact on the resulting model. The question of best or second best never actually comes up in the iteration.

Forward-backward regression accomplishes both first one and then the other, iteratively, so that it is "adding and trimming, adding and trimming" or alternatively asking which is better, adding one or subtracting one in a stepwise fashion, until a stopping point is reached. It suffers from the same limitation as "forward." Most of the time, all three approaches will result in the same sequence of variables in the same order, but not necessarily. Forward stepwise has the advantage that it can always be used, even when the number of subjects is smaller than the number of potential variables, whereas backward stepwise can't.

Best subset regression actually evaluates every possible combination of variables, identifying the combination that gives the lowest error. Best subset regression at first sounds like the best—it is actually picking the subset of variables that works best—but it has two important limitations: first, it is picking the best FROM THIS DATASET, which may not be generalizable; second, it can only be performed on a dataset with a small number of variables (perhaps up to 40, but be prepared to wait) because of the complexity of the calculations.

7.2.4.2   Shrinkage Methods

Instead of actually deleting variables, it is possible to ask the computer to just use "part" of each variable, according to how good it is [6]. The formal term to describe this is a **penalty function**. This is accomplished by adding an additional term to the previous sum of squared residuals, both terms containing the coefficients being optimized. This creates, in essence, a "yin-yang" effect, simultaneously subtracting and adding, which limits the size of the coefficients. For our purposes, understanding the math is far less important than that each variable is shrunk by a specified amount instead of deleting any, as described in Hastie [6].

The earliest approach to shrinkage was named **ridge regression**. Looking at the formula, the trade-off is visible:

$$\beta\text{-ridge} = \text{argmin}_\beta \left[\Sigma(y - \hat{y})^2 + \lambda\Sigma\beta^2 \right]$$

in which **argmin** means finding the values of the coefficients which minimize the argument inside the brackets, and the terms inside the brackets are the SSR and the squared penalty function with a "shrinkage factor-β." B is the vector of coefficients, which is contained in the fact that $\hat{y} = Bx$. So increasing β in the left term of the minimization causes the right term to increase. "λ," the ridge coefficient, is selected by repetitive trial and error to give the most desirable shrinkage pattern. In ridge regression, ALL of the variables remain in the model, but only pieces of each. This requires determining a theoretical number of degrees of freedom, but the software can do that. (For those interested, ridge regression can also be formulated as a process of performing a principle component analysis and a multiple regression simultaneously.) A possible disadvantage of ridge regression is that it doesn't actually remove any variables. This is offset by the fact that it "effectively" reduces the dimensionality PLUS it creates a new set of orthogonal variables that are independent and not correlated. So ridge regression is a way to address dimensionality, independence, and multicollinearity. Ridge regression can be found in a number of R packages, with a relatively user-friendly version in {R:MASS:lm.ridge}.

A more recent approach to shrinkage is known as **lasso** [6]. Lasso combines the general approach of penalized regression with a "cutoff" value, which forces some of the coefficients to zero value, effectively deleting them from the model:

$$\beta\text{lasso} = \text{argmin}\beta_{Ni} \left\{ \Sigma(\hat{y} - \beta x)^2 + \lambda\Sigma|\beta| \right\}$$

subject to $\Sigma|\beta j| \leq t$.

While the penalty in ridge regression is the sum of the squared coefficients, the penalty in lasso is the sum of the absolute values. In the case of lasso, the "yin-yang" is between the sum of SQUARED residuals and the sum of NOT SQUARED absolute values, constrained so that the sum of the absolute value of the coefficients is less than some value "t." The constraint is what forces some of the coefficients to be zero. So the result will be different (and nonlinear). Keep in mind that the goal of modeling is to find the model that works best, defined as performing best on a new set of data (generalizing). Sometimes ridge regression works best and other times lasso. Both methods should be in the toolbox. Lasso can be found at {R:lars:lars}.

Even more recently, **least angle regression** (LAR) [6] evolved from its ridge-lasso origins. LAR is a modified form of lasso but with an important difference—it combines penalization with a stepwise entry of variables based on their correlation with the residuals. Unlike stepwise multiple regression (previously discussed), which enters ALL of a variable, one at a time, LAR enters a portion of a variable, one at a time. This method thus introduces a slightly different approach to dimensionality and adds yet another tool to the toolbox. It is calculated at the same time as the lasso using {R:lars:lars}.

A quick Internet search will demonstrate that new variations of ridge, lasso, LAR, and others are being introduced almost weekly into CRAN. This suggests that the problem of failed assumptions is being addressed slowly, step by step, with each step an additional improvement over traditional multiple regression. Nevertheless it is worth repeating that it seems best to try them all and pick the one that works.

7.2.4.3 Methods That Create New Input Variables

As just described, shrinkage methods penalize the sum of squares by adding in another term, allowing "pieces" of each variable to be included in the model. Another approach is to first transform the variables to eliminate collinearity using principle component regression (PCR) or partial least square regression (PLSR). The shrinkage methods just described can be thought of as combining two mathematical components into a single process. PCR and PLSR split them up, performing an initial conversion of the data into a new set of variables and then following with a multiple regression using the new variables. **PCR** applies an initial principal component analysis (PCA) [7] on only the input variables to construct the new variables and "prioritizes" the new variables based on their eigen values, reducing dimensionality by allowing relatively small contributors to be deleted. Another way to think of this is that the total variance of just the input variables can be repartitioned into a set of orthogonal components, assigning sequentially less of the variance in each subsequent component. This is followed by traditional multiple regression using the new inputs. Keeping all of the principal components addresses non-independence and collinearity; using only some also addresses dimensionality. A limitation of PCR is that it muddies the water if the goal is to understand the role of the input variables, as it creates a new set of variables made up by (loaded) various amounts of the original variables, obscuring the original variables. However, it is not uncommon for the loading of the original variables onto the new variables to "uncover" a deeper level of understanding of the actual "drivers" behind the original dataset.

Partial least square regression (PLSR) also creates new variables, but it uses both the input variables and the outcome variable. After standardizing the original variables to make them more "combinable," and taking into consideration the strength of the relationship between each input and the outcome, a new set of orthogonal variables is created sequentially, basically performing a univariate regression repeatedly, one variable at a time. Unlike PCR, which only considers the total **input** variance in creating the new variables, PLSR focuses on the portion of the variance that is explained by the relationships with the outcome variable in creating the new variables. In other words, while PCR creates new variables based on the variance of only the inputs, PLSR creates new variables based on the actual mean squared residuals.

PLSR is particularly useful in situations where a very large number of measurements are derived from a process, many or most of which don't contribute to the model. PLSR essentially ignores most of the (non-contributing) data and only considers variables that relate to the outcome. PLSR often produces the smallest dimensionality in a very compact model that still includes almost all of the meaningful input information. Minitab has a built-in function for PLSR. PLSR can be found in "R" package **pls** and others [8]. Is PLSR better than PCR? No, just different and sometimes one works better than the other, so both belong in the toolbox.

7.2.4.4   Regression Methods with "Count" Data as Outcome

The prior regression methods used a continuous outcome variable [9]. Often, the outcome variable "counts" something. While there can be a very large number of outcome possibilities, they are constrained to whole numbers. Not the limited number of outcomes we will see in categorical classification models, just whole numbers. It may be tempting to apply multiple regression, but consider trying to interpret 4.3 wound infections! Count data follow what is known as a Poisson distribution. The number of wound infections occurring per unit time is a Poisson variable, as is number of readmissions, number of pulmonary emboli, etc. As the number of counts increases (>30), the Poisson distribution begins to approximate the normal distribution, slowly meeting by about $n = 100$. When the range of the outcome is less than 100, using an ordinary regression model for an outcome that can only take whole number values can give incorrect results. Two methods are available for addressing this: **Poisson regression** and **negative binomial regression**. The two are similar with one very important difference—a Poisson variable MUST pass the test that the mean value is equal to the variance (using descriptive statistics). When this condition is not met, the Poisson regression model is referred to as "over-dispersed," meaning that the variance is larger than the model wants. In such cases the negative binomial, which allows wider variance, is more appropriate. Both methods are supported in R (Poisson regression is found in glm{stats} using family="poisson," and the negative binomial in glm.nb{MASS}),and extensive supporting information, including worked examples, is available by searching for "cran poisson regression" or "cran negative binomial regression."

7.2.4.5   Methods That Use Separating Hyperplanes Instead of Classical Regression

The methods already discussed have all relied on some approach to conducting a regression. An entirely new approach was introduced by Vapnik in the 1960s based on a concept known as maximum separating hyperplanes [10] (Fig. 7.1). A separating hyperplane (or hypertube, which extends beyond three dimensions) can most easily be visualized in its three-dimensional application as the smallest tubular structure that contains the data. This tubular structure has a central "axis" and a radius.

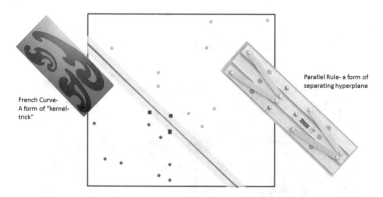

Fig. 7.1 Support vector machine (parallel rules and French curves)

The axis has an associated equation orienting it in space and the radius is described by a sufficient number of vectors extending from the central axis to define the outer surface. These radially oriented vectors are known as support vectors. Instead of having a regression line, based on minimizing variation in a parametric relationship, the nonparametric support vector complex is the minimum hypertube that sufficiently contains the data.

Support vector regression—SVR (R:svm{e1071}) was introduced in 1995 after having already been established as a method for classification (which will be discussed later) in the 1960s. The method identifies the "best" separating hypertube, while allowing "outliers" or even nonlinearity. Since it uses a somewhat "heretical" approach (regression was the accepted mechanism for over 100 years!), it hasn't been widely used, but it has many redeeming qualities making it often superior to regression with its attendant assumptions.

SVR "balances" outliers by defining a "price" for ignoring each outlier and establishing a limit for the total cost, making it possible to pre-establish user-defined limits which "tune" the model. In addition, nonlinear situations can be addressed using SVR with what is known as "the kernel trick." The kernel trick is conceptually complicated, so suffice it to say that it allows a variety of nonlinear models to be constructed. Conceptually, the kernel trick is analogous to a "pantograph," a drawing device that allows tracing one figure and simultaneously recreating a larger or smaller version through a system of interconnected bars (Fig. 7.2). A pantograph typically has a "linear" connection, whereas kernel functions can be other mathematical relationships. There are many kernels that are built into svm software. Which kernel to use can be a challenge, but the goal is simply to find the one that works the best, by trying a few and measuring how well they work. Common kernels are polynomials, radial basis functions, and sigmoidal functions. In essence these are performing "curve fitting" to adjust the hypertube. Mean squared error for each constructed model allows comparing several kernel options as well as traditional regression.

Unlike least square regression (which "is what it is"), optimizing an SVM requires "tuning." Tuning means iteratively varying one or more parameters,

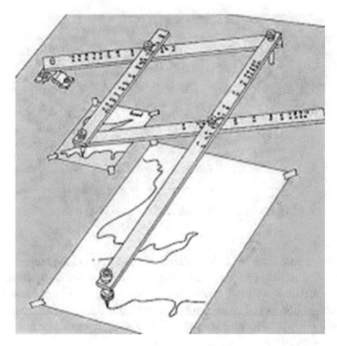

Fig. 7.2 The "kernel trick." The kernel trick is analogous to a "pantograph"; a mechanical device that allows transferring a design from one place to another in a larger or smaller format, based on controllable but definite relationships. Items in one location are simultaneously transmitted to a second location, using the defined relationship but without any calculations

selecting the model that minimizes the mean square error (MSE). In "R," tuning can be accomplished by including it as a component in the svm-syntax or by a "**wrapper**" function called "tune." An extensive discussion of the specifics of svm and svr is available in Hamel [10].

7.2.4.6 Summary of Model Building Concepts/Approaches

Since we have addressed a large amount of dense and perhaps confusing information, it may help to simplify and summarize. Multiple regression, the traditional approach to modeling data with a continuous outcome, is limited by its unavoidable assumptions. Sometimes violating these assumptions results in "bad" models that don't generalize well; yet on the surface they appear "tight" and attractive. To address these limitations, three distinct parametric regression approaches have been developed: subset selection, shrinkage, and new variables. In any given situation one or the other may address the limitations better, and the "best" should be selected. SVR provides a nonparametric approach to regression which largely avoids ALL of the limiting assumptions, leaving only dimensionality as a "demon." A thoughtful approach to creating a regression model should include, at a minimum, multiple regression, a shrinkage method, a hybrid method, and SVR. While the different modeling approaches may be comparable, often one approach clearly stands out as superior based on how well it generalizes to new data.

7.2.4.7   Summary of Regression Methods

Modern regression methods have been developed to address the many limiting assumptions of classical regression. These include approaches to address/modify the input variables by selection, shrinkage, or creating new variables; methods that model count data; and methods that avoid least squares completely by determining a nonparametric hypertube. All methods utilize some method to achieve a "best fit" of the data to some analytical format [6] (Fig. 7.3). Additional new regression methods will continue to be developed, either to further address assumption-based limitations or to focus on a particular type of analytical situation. For the present, the methods presented here should be more than sufficient to allow the thoughtful

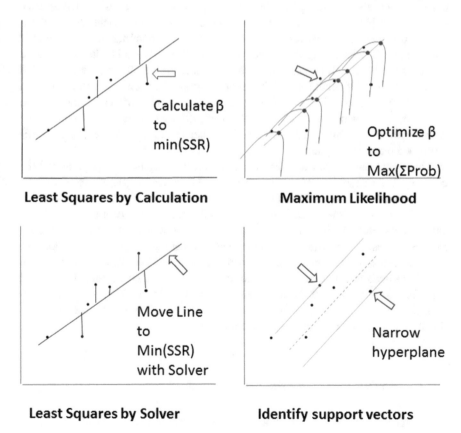

Fig. 7.3 Methods for "best fit" in regression. (**a**) Least squares by calculation; (**b**) maximum likelihood; (**c**) least squares by solver; (**d**) identify support vectors

individual to find and apply a method that works well by being both "tight" (reproducible) and accurate (generalizable). The prudent analyst will approach regression problems with a toolbox of modern tools and a way to identify which is "best."

7.3 Supervised Learning with a Categorical Outcome: Classification

7.3.1 Setting the Stage

Many aspects of modern medical care have discrete outcomes: number of stents placed during a coronary intervention, lived or died, was readmitted or wasn't, developed a wound infection or not, etc. While fundamentally similar to regression, these questions require **discrete**, **categorical** answers rather than a measure of central tendency and a range. Much of the time, the outcome is not only categorical and discrete, but also more specifically **binary** (typically 0,1 as in lived/died). Classification [6] with discrete outcomes requires different approaches from regression, approaches that constrain the predicted outcomes to values between 0 and 1. An example is determining the expected number of postoperative deaths in a case mix of patients. This is accomplished by summing the likelihood (predicted value between 0 and 1) of death for each patient undergoing an operation, estimated from a classification model. This sum (the total expected number of deaths) can then be compared to the actual number of deaths, typically by calculating the ratio of the actual number of deaths to the predicted number (an observed-to-expected (O/E) ratio) as a measure of quality.

The recent enthusiasm for outcome research in medicine has popularized the concept of classification. More specifically, it has made people aware of logistic regression models. But logistic regression is only one of many methods that can be applied to create a classification model. By definition, a classification model has a categorical (often binary) outcome, instead of a continuous outcome, as in regression. But classification can also include methods that have more than two possible outcomes, such as the Linnaean classification system in biology. So while this is an oversimplification, there are two basic approaches to classification: hierarchical classification trees and analytical classification models (analogous to those discussed in regression). In between is an intermediate set of methods based on conditional probability and Bayes' theorem (Fig. 7.4).

7.3.2 Hierarchical Classification

Hierarchical classification using trees has some practical advantages: it is not influenced by nonlinearity, it is well suited to categorical input variables, and the results are easy to explain. The important consideration that characterizes a hierarchical

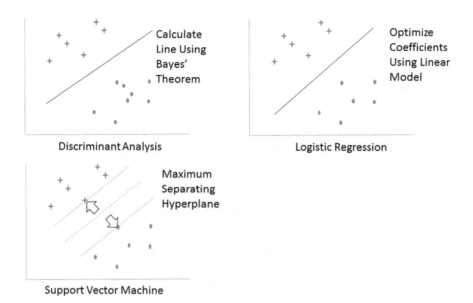

Fig. 7.4 Methods for classification. (**a**) Discriminant analysis (DA), (**b**) logistic regression (LR); (**c**) support vector machine (SVM). Classification models separate data into groups. Note that small changes in the data can substantially alter the line for DA or LR. DA and LR will give different lines. SVM is not altered except by points on lines (support vectors)

classification model is that it has to be **mutually exclusive and exhaustive** (**MEE**)—every item to be classified must be able to be put into one and only one category. An easy solution to the problem of putting each item in some classification is to create a category called "other." This guarantees that all items will be classified, but if too many are placed into "other," the classification model loses its usefulness. The result of a classification tree is that every item will be placed in some bucket, as opposed to an analytical approach which actually creates a continuous outcome, constrained between 0 and 1, which is then dichotomized by rounding up or down.

The usual explanation of a **hierarchical** classification tree is an upside-down branching system, with a small number of "nodes" at the top (typically a single grouping) that each divides into two or more subbranches, continuing until every individual item is accounted for. A horizontal "dividing line" is then established (based on judgment) that creates the "right" number of "buckets" to be useful. The division at each branching is accomplished by minimizing the amount of **entropy** (randomness) at that branch. You probably learned about entropy in high school or college. Entropy is a quantitative expression of randomness; the more random, the greater the entropy. In optimizing a branching split, the goal is to MINIMIZE the randomness which is the same as saying maximize the amount of order or structure. Three common (and related) measures of randomness are entropy, GINI index, and misclassification, which can be used interchangeably as they actually give the same conclusion. It is only important to know that in order to effect a branching split, it is necessary to use some measurement to minimize the randomness. More advanced approaches to hierarchical branching classification trees can then apply additional, probability-based structure to the branching or to "invent" levels in between existing levels (hidden layers) to artificially establish a layer that "makes sense" in creating the structure. Often hierarchical classification trees perform very well in making order out of apparent chaos, enhancing understanding of a set of data, especially when the data are nominal variables, which can be separated into MEE categories, and which have counts/frequencies. Minitab does not have a hierarchical classification method, but methods can be found in R:{rpart} and {tree}.

7.3.3   Models Based on Bayesian (Conditional) Probability

A probability-based approach to classification into categories (Bayesian classification) utilizes conditional probability. If all of the required data are available and the category probabilities are all independent, this is a straightforward application of Bayes' theorem:

$$P(Y \mid X) = P(X \mid Y) \times P(Y) / P(X)$$

So, for example, knowing that (1) all patients with clinical Zollinger-Ellison syndrome (severe, atypical peptic ulcers, marked gastric hyperacidity, and non-Beta islet-cell tumor of the pancreas) have an elevated chromogranin level ($P(C \mid Z) = 100\%$); (2) the incidence of ZES, $P(Z)$, is less than 1/40,000; and (3) the probability of an elevated chromogranin level, $P(C)$, (very low incidence of pancreatic endocrine tumors), is largely due to the false positive rate of 1/40 (2.5% based on the right tail of a normal curve), allows the determination of the probability of ZES given an elevated chromogranin level, $P(Z \mid C)$. Note that this is a largely "deterministic" approach—if all of the necessary elements are present, the result can be calculated.

More likely, however, is that the data are not "complete" and the actual probabilities are not known to be independent, but require some level of inference. Methods have been developed that include "leaps of faith" in the independence of the likelihoods. A moderate leap uses "naïve Bayesian classification" and a giant leap, a "Bayesian Belief Network." Both are supported in "R" {R:e1071:naiveBayes, and (R:bnlearn) [11].

7.3.4   Models Based on a Measure of Proximity
(Distance or Similarity)

Another modeling method for classification involves assigning subjects to groups based on some measure of "proximity" rather than on the basis of probability or entropy. As mentioned previously, proximity measures can be based either on an actual distance or a measure of similarity. One such distance-based method is known as **k-nearest neighbor (knn) classification**. Instead of using a statistical dimension to define a class, *k*-nearest neighbor establishes a region for each class defined by a specified number of points in the training set closest to each point in the test set. The "fit" is optimized by evaluating the model using different values of "k". knn classification can be found in a number of R packages: **class**, **knn**, **kknn**, and **FNN**. In each case, there is no actual model calculated. Rather, R proceeds through the test set, looks at the "k" closest points in the training set and "votes" on which class the point belongs to. Note that Knn methods are susceptible to unbalanced datasets.

7.3.5   Model-Based Classification Methods

Discussing "Classification" often triggers "logistic regression" although **logistic regression** was not the earliest approach or necessarily the best approach to model-based classification, and many advanced methods have been developed to address the limitations and assumptions of logistic regression (very much as we have already learned in multiple regression). The earliest approach to model-based classification applied ordinary linear regression using the binary outcome variable as a continuous variable. While this occasionally works, it is severely limited in that the outcome is unconstrained, and there is no way to properly interpret a probability greater than 1.0 or a negative probability. Since so many computer methods are now available, there is no good reason to "force" linear regression to do classification.

   Linear discriminant analysis—LDA (or simply discriminant analysis) was the earliest approach to constrain the range of the outcome variable. It applies Bayes' theorem by assuming that the class conditional probabilities (sensitivity) are Gaussian with a shared covariance matrix (essentially uniform variance). The method can actually be calculated on a slide rule, so it antedates modern computers (Fisher-1936). A menu-driven method can be found in Minitab {Stat:Multivariate: DiscriminantAnalysis} as well as in R (Mass(lda)). It has the big advantage that it works for greater than two classes of outcomes, so it should definitely be tried in these cases. The assumptions of normality and single covariance matrix are limiting but usually not crippling. Modern computers can handle situations where the covariance matrices are not the same with a method called Quadratic Discriminant Analysis, similarly available in most modern software (R:MASS(qda)). Although "old," discriminant analysis still belongs in the toolbox.

   Logistic regression (McFadden-1973) evolved from studies of population growth going back to the 1800s, known as the **logistic** ($\log[\exp(x)/(1+\exp(x)]$). The logistic is simply the log of a probability calculated from odds ($P = \text{Odds} / (1 + \text{Odds})$. The logistic is strictly constrained between 0 and 1, plus the central portion is very similar in shape to a normal distribution. Ongoing use led to the development of a related function, the **logit** ($\log[\exp(x)/(1-\exp(x)]$). Recalling that $x/(1-x)$ represents odds, the logit is simply **log-odds**.

LDA simply applies conditional probability. Logistic regression differs from LDA by setting the odds ratio equal to a linear equation and solving for the coefficients. In other words, the input variables form the equation of a straight line in x. The input variables, then, are subject to the same assumptions as in linear regression: additivity, linearity, normality of the residuals, and uniformity of variance.

Unlike LDA, which can easily handle more than two classes, logistic regression is most straightforward with two, ideally suited to a binary outcome. More than two categories is accomplished by multiple pairwise analysis and comparing the results. But more than two outcomes is possible, and Minitab includes a menu-driven option {Stat:Regression:OrdinalLogisticRegression}. But logistic regression utilizes iterative likelihood maximization, so the solution often takes a long time or may never "converge" to a solution. One classification category is arbitrarily set as the comparator, so in a binary classification there is only one actual equation, making it analytically straight forward. The resulting expression <u>for the binary case</u> is

$$\log\left(\frac{P(G=0 \mid X=x)}{P(G=1 \mid X=x)}\right) = \beta_0 + \beta_k X \quad (X = input\, matrix)$$

which converts into the form

$$P(G=0 \mid X=x) = \exp(\beta_0 + \beta_k X) / (1 + \exp(\beta_0 + \beta_k X))$$

and

$$P(G=1 \mid X=x) = 1 / (1 + \exp(\beta_0 + \beta_k X)).$$

(I include the equations because they are usually included in a "help" result.)

The resulting probabilities for class $=(0)$ or (1) are both constrained between 0 and 1 and together add up to 1, forcing the classification to be one or the other. The actual calculations use an iterative optimization process, often requiring a very large number of iterations. Like its cousin, linear regression, logistic regression requires a careful understanding of the input variables. Subset selection is the most common method, methods comparable to those previously discussed in regression are available: shrinkage (ridge logistic regression in R:logisticRidge [12], new variables (principle components followed by logistic regression, etc.). As in multiple regression, these modern variations often give a better solution by addressing multicollinearity and dimensionality.

Although it is often thought that the assignment to one class or the other in these methods is "clean," in fact it is simply that if $P \leq 0.5$ it is assigned to class (0) and if $P > 0.5$ to class(1). A difference of, say, 1 % could change the result! Many of the methods provide an output that includes the actual probabilities for each record (such as fuzzy classification in R). Careful assessment of the actual calculated likelihoods will demonstrate if a large number of records are actually "in the middle."

7.3.6   Other Classification Methods

Although LDA and logistic regression have been the workhorses of classification and are still quite useful, newer approaches have been introduced to address the limitations of the assumptions and to provide alternative models which may perform better. All of the techniques described in the section on regression have been adapted to classification models including **ridge classification** [13], **lasso classification** [14], **principle component classification (perform PCA on inputs, then logistic regression)**, and **partial least squares discriminant analysis** [15]. **SVM** [10] were originally described for classification and frequently work better than regression-based methods.

Ridge classification and Lasso classification can be accomplished by setting the outcome class in the training set to -1 and $+1$ and utilizing the corresponding approach previously described in "regression." As in regression, ridge will shrink all of the input variables by varying amounts, whereas lasso will force some of the variables to zero (deleting them) and shrink the others. When applied to a validation set or new set of data, negative values and positive values assign the two categories.

Partial least squares discriminant analysis (R:plsda{muma}) was developed specifically for very high dimensionality situations where most of the data are not contributing to the model, so it focuses on narrow segments of the data. It typically results in substantial dimensionality reduction, often to just a few remaining variables, without loss of contributing data.

As mentioned, support vector machines (svm) were originally created as classification methods, based on the **maximum separating hyperplane**. Unlike support vector regression, which defines a hypertube that includes the data, svm for classification creates a hypertube that separates the data. Since svm isn't based on regression, it is not model-based in the usual sense and is distribution-free. As in the regression application of svm, a cost function can be used to allow misclassification and a kernel function (polynomial, radial basis, or sigmoidal) can be used for nonlinear models. A svm must be "tuned," as described in svr.

References

1. Kutner MH, Nachtsheim C, Neter J. Applied linear regression models. 4th ed. New York: McGraw-Hill; 2004. 701 p.
2. Poole MA, O'Farrell PN. The assumptions of the linear regression model. Trans Inst Br Geogr. 1971;52:145–58.
3. Anscombe FJ. Graphs in statistical analysis. Am Stat. 1973;27(1):17–21.
4. Newton I. Minitab Cookbook. Birmingham: Packt Publishing; 2014.
5. Hastie T, James G, Tibshirani R, Witten D. An introduction to statistical learning: with applications in R. New York: Springer; 2013.
6. Hastie T, Friedman JH, Tibshirani R. The elements of statistical learning: data mining, inference, and prediction. 2, corrected 7 printing edth ed. New York: Springer; 2009.
7. Jolliffe IT. Principal component analysis, vol. xiii. New York: Springer; 1986. 271 p.

8. Benneyan J, Lloyd R, Plsek P. Statistical process control as a tool for research and healthcare improvement. Qual Saf Health Care. 2003;12(6):458–64.
9. Jewell N, Hubbard A. Modelling counts. The Poisson and negative binomial regression, Analysis of longitudinal studies in epidemiology. Boca Raton: Chapman & Hall; 2006.
10. Hamel LH. Knowledge discovery with support vector machines. New York: Wiley; 2011.
11. Scutari M. Learning Bayesian networks with the bnlearn R package. arXiv preprint arXiv:09083817. 2009.
12. Askin RG, Standridge CR. Modeling and analysis of manufacturing systems, vol. xvi. New York: Wiley; 1993. 461 p.
13. Loh W-L. Linear discrimination with adaptive ridge classification rules. J Multivar Anal. 1997;62(2):169–80.
14. Ghosh D, Chinnaiyan AM. Classification and selection of biomarkers in genomic data using LASSO. J Biomed Biotechnol. 2005;2005(2):147–54.
15. Westerhuis JA, Hoefsloot HC, Smit S, Vis DJ, Smilde AK, van Velzen EJ, et al. Assessment of PLSDA cross validation. Metabolomics. 2008;4(1):81–9.

Chapter 8
Unsupervised Machine Learning: Datasets Without Outcomes

Scenario

Dr. Ralph Williams is the chief of clinical chemistry at Westshore Medical Center. The Chief Financial Officer has determined that Westshore physicians order at least twice as many laboratory tests since they were given the ability to create their own order sets. Williams has been charged with analyzing all of the apparent order sets, their frequencies, and their importance. Although the new computer system is state of the art, it doesn't actually allow analyzing the order sets themselves, so he has to use the actual laboratory database to determine which laboratory tests were ordered at the same time. He uses association analysis with a software method called "arules" in a powerful software system called "R." He identifies the 20 most frequent order sets and, using these data, merges with an outcome database to determine if there is any apparent impact on clinical outcome.

8.1 Unsupervised Learning: Models Without Outcomes

Regression and classification models are very popular, particularly in outcome studies. However, there are occasions when there isn't an appropriate outcome variable: there really isn't a definite outcome variable, there are several potential outcome variables, or it is desirable to analyze the model first for enhanced understanding before defining an outcome variable. **Association analysis** and **clustering** are powerful methods that achieve these goals. While currently underutilized in the medical literature, both families of methods can provide comprehensive understanding of the structure of a dataset as well as an initial analysis of what goes with what. Association analysis is ideal for analyzing datasets which include what might be called "transactions," sets of things that have names (nominal variables) with their

© Springer International Publishing Switzerland 2016

P.J. Fabri, *Measurement and Analysis in Transforming Healthcare Delivery*,

DOI 10.1007/978-3-319-40812-5_8

frequencies of occurrence, often referred to as "marketbaskets." Cluster analysis is best suited for quantitative data without an outcome or for which analysis is desired independent of the outcome to determine structure and relationships. The concept of a "training set" has no meaning in unsupervised learning methods, so there is no method of assessing the success of an analysis except in relative terms, compared to another method. All conclusions are inferences.

8.2   Unsupervised Learning with Nominal Data: Association Analysis

8.2.1   Setting the Stage

The widespread availability of computers in healthcare has allowed the accumulation of large databases which are now "mature." Since "meaningful" outcome data were infrequently included in these collections, they consist primarily of names, counts, and measures of "things." Useful information can be developed from these data, allowing a better understanding of the activities and their relationships during the care cycle. Examples of such datasets include preoperative laboratory tests, medications used in a cardiology ward, personal hygiene products used in bedside care, etc. Enhanced understanding of such processes can lead to improved utilization, better education and training, more meaningful outcome measures, etc. Genome-wide studies (sets of single-nucleotide polymorphisms (SNP), etc.) as well as genetic trait analyses [1] (sets of character traits or sets of genes associated with a trait) are particularly well suited to association analysis. Another example could be analyzing all of the laboratory test orders for a year to determine what combinations are commonly ordered together. In fact, much of hospital-level data are actually collections of "transactions." While they may be able to be "linked" with outcome data from other data sources, the hospital datasets themselves usually don't contain them.

8.2.2   Terminology in Association Analysis

Of all of the analytical methods discussed in this volume, association analysis is conceptually the simplest, consisting almost exclusively of identifying which items or sets of items are frequent (called frequent itemsets), how frequent they are (support), and how interesting they are (confidence and lift). (Perhaps this simplicity explains why association analysis is so rarely used in the medical literature.) Examples of frequent itemsets might be preoperative laboratory tests, hospital bills, operating room supply orders, etc. The healthcare world is full of datasets of transactions. Although analyzing transaction datasets is straightforward, the terminology can appear confusing.

For the typical transaction dataset, since there is a very large number of available items, a spreadsheet contains a large number of zeroes (things that were NOT ordered, purchased, etc.), which are actually "empty." A dataset with a large number of empty cells is referred to as a **sparse dataset**. Consider for example the large number of potential items that are NOT purchased in a trip to the grocery store, about which no thought was given while in the store. Or laboratory tests that are NOT ordered on a particular patient on a particular day. A decision NOT to do something is quite different from not even considering doing it—the former is a decision, the latter only a happenstance. Sparse datasets often do not behave well analytically and usually require adaptations in analysis to handle the sparseness. It is important to recognize a sparse dataset and be prepared to take precautions [2].

A collection of one or more items is referred to as an **itemset**. In a dataset with only 8 different available items, a collection of all possible itemsets includes each combination of 1, 2, 3 … 8 items, 256 in total, unless order is important in which case the number of permutations is 40,320. Typically, however, only a small number of these combinations occur frequently, and these are known as the **frequent itemsets**. Enumerating the frequent itemsets first requires a decision as to how frequent is frequent. This can be accomplished by listing all of the existing itemsets with their absolute and relative frequencies, or there may be selected defined minimum number of items.

The next question to ask is how often does Y occur, given that X has occurred. This creates an **association rule** notated as $X \to Y$ and read "if X, then Y." The left side, X, is referred to as the **precedent** or **antecedent** and Y, the **consequent**. The often-quoted textbook example asks if a husband is sent to a convenience store to buy milk and diapers, what is the most likely third item (answer—beer), so X is an itemset {diapers, milk} and Y is {beer} written {diapers, milk} $\to$ {beer}. But anything that CONTAINS the itemset (e.g., {diapers, milk, beer}) is ALSO an itemset. Association analysis software can enumerate ALL of the itemsets or just the frequent itemsets if "frequent" is defined. The relative frequency of a particular itemset (as percent of total transactions) is referred to as its **support**, where support is defined as the number of records that contain that specific combination of items (plus larger itemsets that also contain it) divided by the total number of transactions. In other words, support is the percentage of all transactions that contain a specific combination of items within a "purchase" of whatever size. The next question is "How important/interesting is this." The term **confidence** is used to express interest—of all of the transactions that contain X, what percentage contain both X and Y. In looking at a pre-procedure battery of laboratory tests, X might be CBC plus basic metabolic panel, and Y might be coagulation studies. We are interested in how often coags are ordered together with CBC and BMP. The support is what percentage of pre-procedure laboratory orders contain all three. The confidence is what percentage of the orders containing CBC and BMP also contain coags, which is equivalent to the support of the combination of all three divided by the support of only the first two. In probability terminology, support is $P(X,Y)$—probability of X and Y—and confidence is $P(Y|X)$—probability of Y given X. A third component of a typical association analysis involves determination of **lift**. Lift is defined as the confidence of an association rule (combination of items X and Y) divided by the expected confidence, but mathematically it is simply the support of the combination X and Y divided by the support of X and the support of Y, and represents the multiple of the likelihood of random chance—a lift greater than 1 means more likely than by chance and the larger the lift, the more so.

In equation form:

$$\text{Support}(X \rightarrow Y) = f(X \text{ and } Y) / N$$

$$\text{Confidence}(X \rightarrow Y) = f(X \text{ and } Y) / f(X)$$

$$\text{Lift}(X \rightarrow Y) = f(X \text{ and } Y) / f(X) f(Y), \text{where } f(\ ) \text{ is the frequency}$$

If the frequency of X and Y was no greater than would be expected from the individual probabilities of X and Y, the lift would be 1. If X and Y occur together more frequently than would be expected from their individual frequencies, the lift is greater than 1 as a function of how much more likely. Since "X" is a list of things and "Y" is a single item, the lift only addresses that specific rule and not the other permutations of those items.

The analysis of a transaction-type dataset usually needs to be focused by establishing a minimum level of support that is "meaningful," a minimum level of confidence that "is interesting," and a minimum level of lift or "how interesting." As previously mentioned, in the absence of an "outcome" it is not possible to define "how good" or "how important," only "how interesting." And it obviously can't be used to assess cause and effect. A quantitative expression of degree of association can be estimated by several methods, none of which meets all aspects of "how interesting," but combining a few of these should offer a useful interpretation [3].

Datasets appropriate for association analysis include NOMINAL variables (things), and the only mathematical operator that makes sense involves counting. The square root of the number of CBCs is computationally possible but conceptually meaningless. So why would one do association analysis? The simple answer is that association analysis is sometimes the only analytic method that is appropriate. A more thoughtful response might be that to improve something requires measuring it. Without understanding what IS, it is impossible to make it better.

Typical menu-driven software packages don't have methods for association analysis. R provides methods in the package "arules" (apriori{arules}}, eclat{arules}), and "arulesViz" (plot{arulesViz}), as well as packages specifically designed for genome and genetic analyses. "apriori" and "eclat" are two slightly different approaches to association analysis and should be thought of as complementary, with eclat often being more efficient. "eclat" produces a list of itemsets selected based on levels of support and confidence. "apriori" can be "asked" (called "coerced") to provide an output of all of the itemsets that meet a user-defined set of criteria (the antecedent is known as "lhs" and the consequent "rhs" and can be specified). It can also be "coerced" to provide the association rules. "arulesViz" contains a very useful plot function that provides visualization of itemsets, support, and lift to assist in selecting cutoffs in support and confidence. Both apriori and eclat can produce either itemset output (class "itemset") or rules (class "rules") with corresponding formats.

Infrequent itemsets—Although it is usual to identify frequent itemsets from a transaction set, sometimes a more interesting approach is to look for things that are "uncommon." That is, identifying outliers may be more interesting than identifying what is frequent. Specifically itemizing "the bottom" of the support or confidence vector will select out **infrequent itemsets** for further analysis and interpretation.

While apparently often overlooked because of its simplicity, association analysis can provide a deep understanding of the content and relationships in a dataset. More importantly, sometimes it is the ONLY analytical method that is appropriate for a set of data.

8.3 Unsupervised Learning with Quantitative Data: Clustering

8.3.1 Setting the Stage

Hospital and practice databases contain large amounts of quantitative data: laboratory results, operation duration times, turnover times, number of delinquent discharge summaries, locations of highway accidents to identify new helicopter staging sites, etc. Often there isn't a defined outcome variable or perhaps just understanding the groupings or clusters of the data would dramatically enhance understanding of either the problem or the solution. Such problems are the domain of **clustering** [4, 5].

Clustering is a technique of creating groupings of items that are more alike than the others based on a **proximity measure**, which could be a **distance** or a **similarity**. Since there is no "teacher" to evaluate the "correctness" of the groups, success is typically measured by some measure of how "tight" the groups are. Also, since there is typically no prior definition of how many groups, any number of groups is possible. At this point it is critically important to clearly understand that if asked to create a specific number of groups, the computer software <u>will</u> create THAT NUMBER of groups, with no regard to correctness. The optimum number of groups can only be estimated by making a comparison with some external "agent": a theory or premise that states a number of groups, prior published work that established the number of groups, or a measurement of "how good" to compare different potential numbers. But it bears repeating that telling a computer to create four groups WILL create four groups, right or wrong.

There are many potential proximity measures, but typically there is only one or a few that can apply to a specific set of data. Quantitative data are likely to be clustered by a physical distance measurement (L1-Manhattan; L2-Euclidean; etc.). Multidimensional data are often clustered by Mahalanobis distance [4]. Both quantitative and qualitative data might be best clustered by density (the number of datapoints per unit). Datasets with some qualitative data might be best clustered by similarity, for example text data, into what is called a similarity (or dissimilarity) matrix. An alternative way of looking at possible proximities is to consider nominal, ordinal, interval, and ratio data and the types of relevant approaches. In addition to creating a set of groups that are otherwise "at the same layer," it is also possible to create multiple layers by establishing hierarchical clustering, such as parent-child and set-subset. It is even possible to "invent" a **hidden layer** (imaginary, but it seems to add "sense") in creating a hierarchy.

8.3.2   Approaches to Clustering

Algorithms for establishing clusters minimize the sum of the proximities "within" clusters relative to the proximities "between" clusters. **Hierarchical clustering**, the most "democratic method," either starts with everything in one cluster and then successively creates two, three, four, etc. clusters until every datapoint is its own cluster (known as divisive clustering), OR starts with every datapoint as a cluster and successively creates smaller numbers of clusters until all are again in one cluster (agglomerative clustering). **K-nearest-neighbor** (knn) clustering takes a combinatorial approach, trying various values for "k," the number of elements in a cluster. **Expectation-maximization** uses repetitive trial and error to optimize the location of a parametric distribution to create clusters by minimizing the sum of squared residuals. **K-means**, the workhorse of clustering, determines "k" clusters by minimizing the Euclidean distances. Hierarchical clustering can be performed easily in MiniTab (Stat:Multivariate:ClusterObservations) or RExcel/Rcommander (Statistics:Dimensional Analysis:ClusterAnalysis:HierarchicalClusterAnalysis). It is a useful place to start as it provides a visual assessment of what each number of clusters looks like. **agnes{cluster}** and **diana{cluster}** in "R" provide methods for agglomerative and divisive hierarchical clustering. K-means can be accomplished in MiniTab (Stat:Multivariate:ClusterKmeans) or R (Statistics:Dimensional Analysis:Cluster:KmeansClusterAnalysis) and provides substantial diagnostic information about a specified number of clusters. Leaving RCommander, there are several other methods in R for clustering: Kmeans{stats} in R will iteratively explore a range of "k" and provide the optimum number of clusters. "pam" (partitioning around medioids) in R is probably the most "useful" approach to centroid-based clustering, providing full diagnostic information, but requires defining "k" for each run. **fanny{cluster}** (fuzzy clustering) provides an interesting way to look at clustering, but also reveals a "behind-the-scenes" view of partitioning. Distance-based partitioning actually uses the probability of each point belonging to each of the potential clusters, and then assigns the cluster to the one with the greatest probability, but in most methods these are "rounded off" and assigned a whole cluster number. **fanny** shows these probabilities for each value in each cluster, illuminating the potential problem of "being on the cusp" where a minute change in probability alters the cluster assignment. Stated again, unlike in classification, there is no "correct answer" to assess "how good."

Density-based clustering provides an entirely different approach to creating clusters. Density-based clustering aggregates elements into clusters after selecting levels of density (number of items per unit volume) that correspond to "inside," "outside," or "on the border" of groups. As an example, a "density-based clustering" of the cities in Florida would place Jacksonville, Miami, Orlando, and Tampa (all greater than one million population) in the same cluster, yet Jacksonville and Miami would not be in the same cluster by distance. When it does not appear that "useful" clusters can be identified based on physical distance, a density-based approach should be evaluated. Density-based clustering uses some variation of the DBScan algorithm and can be found in flexible procedures for clustering, dbscan{fpc}. Density-based clustering requires specifying a "decision level" for density expressed as the minimum number of points (minPts) within a specified distance (eps). Once again it requires trial and error to determine optimum values for these parameters. Each point is then assigned to "inside," "outside," and "on the border."

8.3.3   Validating Clusters

Since clustering doesn't include use of a "supervisor," the validity of the clustering process must be assessed by other methods. Two common metrics are useful: clustering tendency and apparent validity.

Estimating clustering tendency involves enumerating two components: the tightness/separation of the clusters and the number of clusters. A common approach to evaluating the **clustering tendency** is to measure the mean square error of the points in the cluster relative to the **centroid** (mathematical center of a cluster set, but not an actual data point) or **medioid** (an actual datapoint that is the closest to the mathematical center). The MSE will decrease in moving from 1 to 2 to 3, etc. clusters until it plateaus for higher numbers of clusters, but the transition can often be gradual, making a selection of optimum number of clusters difficult. A more "obvious" approach, avoiding an often subtle change in MSE, is known as the **silhouette coefficient** or **silhouette index** [4]. The silhouette can be thought of as the size of the "footprint" of a cluster relative to the average distance to the next closest cluster. This method actually consists of repeatedly calculating the distances between each and every point in a cluster and each and every point in every other cluster, which, if done manually, would be a daunting task, but is easily accomplished by a computer. A silhouette can be determined for each value of "k" clusters using the formula

$$\text{Silhouette}\left(C_k\right) = \left\{\left(b(i) - a(i)\right) / \max\left(b(i) \text{ or } a(i)\right)\right\}$$

where $b(i)$ is the average distance (dissimilarity) between clusters and $a(i)$ the average distance (dissimilarity) within a cluster. The silhouette can be calculated for each one of "k" clusters and then averaged. The value of "k" that gives the largest silhouette index is selected as the optimum number of clusters, with a maximum value of 9. Typically a good clustering will give an average silhouette index of 0.75 or better. A graph of silhouette index vs. "k" shows a "spike" at the optimum "k" rather than a transition, making it easier to interpret visually. Three specific partitioning methods within {cluster} (**pam**, **clara**, and **fanny**) contain silhouette as an attribute, callable with **silinfo()** or **$silinfo**. Otherwise, any clustering algorithm can be evaluated with **silhouette(X),** where X is the name of the model (e.g., model1). Silhouette is automatically plotted in some methods, but can be called with plot (X). The graph shows a horizontal bar, made up of horizontal lines for each set of silhouettes, the average silhouette within each cluster to the right, and the overall average silhouette at the bottom. It is the overall silhouette that should be maximized. The silhouette index also serves as a convenient platform for estimating the most appropriate **number of clusters** by selecting the clustering with the largest silhouette.

An additional approach addresses whether the data themselves actually are likely to be clustered. A random set of data points is generated within the data region and a random set is sampled from the actual data. The **Hopkins statistic**, **H** [4], compares the summed distances for a specified number of nearest neighbors in the actual data sample (Σw) with the same number of neighbors in the random set (Σu), using the equation

$$H = \frac{\pounds w}{\pounds u + \pounds w}$$

with values of H ranging from 0 to 1. If the data are "highly clustered," H approaches 1; if the data are distributed in a regular pattern through the data space, 0; and if the actual data are comparable to a random sample, 0.5.

Apparent validity could be assessed either by using external information (which wasn't used in the clustering process) as a "supervisor" (semi-supervised) or by assessing the "face validity" by comparison with known concepts, comparing with other clustering methods, prior research, or SME assessment. If a classification actually existed but was intentionally left out of the clustering to see if the dataset had clusters, comparing the clusters with the actual classification can be accomplished by all of the techniques described previously in **Classification**: entropy, correlation, Jaccard, precision, recall, etc. In either case, in order to be clusters they have to look like clusters! Plotting and visualizing are useful.

Medical datasets often lend themselves to another interesting method of clustering, when a single uniform measurement, such as a patient measure or a laboratory measurement, is made in a large number of patients. Examples include looking at the results of the laboratory test BNP (brain natriuretic peptide) in a large number of patients to see if the values actually correspond to different degrees of congestive heart failure (without specifying them in advance) or looking at diastolic blood pressure in a large number of individuals to determine if there are underlying classes. This powerful clustering-based approach, **expectation-maximization** or **mixture modeling**, requires the assumption that the clusters follow a specified probability distribution function, typically the normal distribution. Since the metrics just mentioned are all of the same measurement in the same units, this might be a reasonable assumption, but the distribution and residuals should still be examined. It might be necessary to identify the correct distribution (for example, lognormal) from the entire dataset first, using Individual Distribution Identification in Minitab. Then, by optimizing the likelihood function as the parameters (for example, mean and variance) are iteratively varied, it is possible to identify the most likely number of underlying groups, as well as their individual means and variances. Such **model-based clustering** can be accomplished using Mclust{mclust} in R. It is important to type the lower case, library(mclust), when loading the package and the upper case (Mclust) when calling the method in R-code. Most typically the univariate mode (as represented by the two examples) and unequal variance are chosen, so the code would be

$$model1 = Mclust(dataset, modelNames = c("E","V"))$$

which instructs R to evaluate both equal and unequal group variances. The output is obtained with "parameters (model1)". Numerous examples can be found in the R-documentation and in the example in (Mclust). Recall that if the sample sizes are "not small" (>30) and the ratio of the largest and smallest variances is less than approximately 1.5, the variances can probably be assumed to be equal (F-test of equality of variances).

Clustering is a very useful tool, both when there is no outcome variable and when it is helpful to "explore" the data to see if there is a match with the existing classification, prior to building a classification model. Since clustering is attempting to identify a true set of categorization, empirically from the data, it is reassuring when the result corresponds with the theory and enlightening when it does not.

References

1. Goldstein DB. Common genetic variation and human traits. N Engl J Med. 2009;360(17):1696.
2. Albinali F, Davies N, Friday A, editors. Structural learning of activities from sparse datasets. Fifth annual IEEE international conference on pervasive computing and communications 2007 PerCom'07. IEEE; 2007.
3. Tan H. Knowledge discovery and data mining. Berlin: Springer; 2012. p. 3–9.
4. Tan PNSM, Kumar V. Introduction to data mining. Boston: Pearson-Addison Wesley; 2006. p. 22–36.
5. Hastie T, Friedman JH, Tibshirani R. The elements of statistical learning: data mining, inference, and prediction. 2, corrected 7 printing edth ed. New York: Springer; 2009.

Chapter 9
Survival Analysis

Scenario

Jim Ferguson is the director of the solid organ transplant program. They now have 40 years of data from their living-related donor kidney transplant registry. Over the decades, newer concepts of immunology, newer rejection medications, and new biomarkers have been introduced into the armamentarium. The Kaplan-Meier actuarial survival curve for the most recent 10-year cohort looks quite different from the cohort of four decades ago. Jim decides to use a log-rank test to compare survival curves and a Cox proportional hazard model to analyze individual factors that might be contributing to the difference. He is reminded by his biostatistician that the Cox model has some important assumptions, so he goes back to the data to determine if the factors of interest are actually proportional and additive.

9.1 Concepts of Survival and Hazard

Many opportunities exist in clinical medicine and in the medical literature for the measurement of survival. For clinicians, the term survival immediately brings to mind patient survival, but the same approach to survival applies to how long until an MRI device fails, an AA-battery lasts, etc. Since these are time measurements, they are characteristically NOT straight lines but rather exponential curves. Also typically, they can usually be converted to a straight line by taking the log.

Survival analysis requires a different approach from the previous analytical methods [1], based on an understanding of the **survival function** and the **hazard function**. In brief, the survival function describes the rate of decrease in percent surviving or functioning at standard intervals over time, and the hazard function describes changes occurring to the survival function along the way. Imagine a probability

© Springer International Publishing Switzerland 2016
P.J. Fabri, *Measurement and Analysis in Transforming Healthcare Delivery*,
DOI 10.1007/978-3-319-40812-5_9

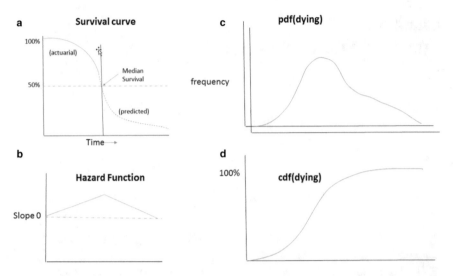

Fig. 9.1 (**a**) Survival curve, (**b**) hazard function, (**c**) probability distribution function (pdf), (**d**) cumulative distribution function (cdf). The survival curve shows the component derived from actual data (*solid*) and the projected component (*dashed*). Immediately below is the hazard function, the rate of change of survival. The pdf shows the point frequency and the cdf the cumulative percentage surviving

distribution function (pdf) showing number of deaths as a function of time, **f(t)**, after a percutaneous coronary intervention. It will start out like a bell-shaped curve with a tail extending to the right, meaning few deaths initially followed by increasing numbers of deaths, which then gradually tapers off over a long time, ending with "high outliers." Summing deaths cumulatively over time produces a cumulative distribution function (cdf) represented as **F(t)**, which starts out at zero and then progressively increases in a sigmoidal fashion until it reaches 100% at some point, crossing the 50th percentile at the value of the median. $1 - F(t)$ is the corresponding survival function, **S(t)**, starting at 100% and decreasing in a curvilinear fashion (if followed long enough) to 0% surviving. The **hazard function** is simply minus the slope of the log of survival. The log straightens the curve, minus inverts the direction (hazard is in the opposite direction of survival!), and the slope indicates the steepness of the change over time. So if survival improves over time there will be a negative hazard function, whereas if the rate of dying escalates, the hazard function will be positive. Only if the log of survival stays constant will the hazard function be zero. Figure 9.1 shows a survival curve (starting at 100% survival and decreasing over time): a hazard function curve (increasing rate of change followed by decreasing; the probability distribution function of death; and the cumulative distribution function of death). Figure 9.2 shows three typical survival curves on the left (left axis) and their hazard functions on the right showing increasing hazard, decreasing hazard, and constant hazard. Trying to sort this out from the survival curves is difficult, whereas examining the hazard functions clearly demonstrates whether the hazard is "worsening," "lessening," or staying the same.

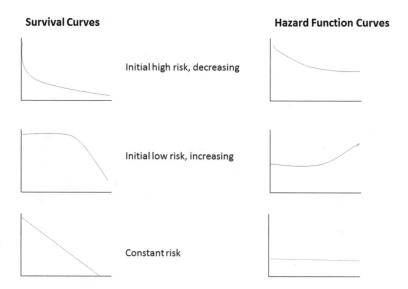

Fig. 9.2 Three different survival curves (*left*) and their corresponding hazard functions (*right*)

9.2   Censoring of Data

Censoring is an important consideration in survival analysis. The term, as used here, indicates simply that there is incomplete information at some point in time for a particular patient. When looking at patient survival, for example, left censoring means that there is missing information BEFORE measurements begin, such as the unknown duration of presence of a disease prior to being diagnosed; right censoring (more common in medical usage) indicates that there is missing information AFTER, such as patients who were alive at last office visit. Implicit in both of these is the definition of a defined "START" – survival after a surgical procedure starts with the procedure (no left censoring, but unless follow-up is VERY long there will be right censoring as some patients will still be alive); survival after identifying a colon cancer at colonoscopy has an uncertain amount of time ON THE LEFT, prior to the colonoscopy, as well as on the right.

9.3   Biases Inherent in Survival Analysis: Lead-Time, Length, and Overdiagnosis Bias

Ascertainment bias (factors influencing WHEN a diagnosis is made) is a "cousin" of censoring and is commonly expressed in three different but related ways: lead-time bias, length bias, and overdiagnosis [2]. **Lead-time bias** is simply a statement that if a disease is diagnosed EARLIER IN ITS COURSE (all other things being equal), people will appear to live longer. An example of that is high-resolution mammography in breast cancer—lesions are diagnosed much earlier than by physical exam, but they're the same lesions. **Length bias** is slightly different in that there is often a tendency for earlier diagnosis to identify abnormalities that have a more favorable outcome (in addition to being diagnosed earlier). This appears also to exist in breast cancer, as newer imaging techniques tend to diagnosis "in situ" lesions. **Overdiagnosis** is a logical extension of the previous two—very early diagnosis can identify "pre" abnormalities that will never actually develop into disease! This may exist for both breast cancer and prostate cancer [3], for example. Diagnostic tests are identifying something much earlier, with an increased likelihood of identifying more favorable lesions. Many of which will actually not develop into a physical malignancy during the patient's lifetime. These biases are important to the analyst because they make identification of a REAL improvement in survival more difficult. As enhanced diagnostic methods are developed, these biases will typically increase. They are manifest when percentage survival appears to be increasing yet the number of individuals dying per 100,000 population remains the same. While this COULD be due to the simultaneous increase in the incidence of the actual disease and an improvement leading to increased survival, the fact that the overall number of people dying remains constant strongly suggests that more individuals are being diagnosed with a category of disease that has a favorable prognosis. This is a rather new understanding in medicine, as traditionally diseases like cancer were thought to always be progressive unless "cured," largely because forms of "predisease" that didn't lead to actual disease would not have been identified!

9.4   Analytical Methods Based on Survival

Armed with the concepts of survival and hazard, three commonly used "survival-based" methods fall naturally into place: calculating actuarial survival (Kaplan-Meier), comparing survival (log-rank), and evaluating contributors to survival (Cox proportional hazards) [4].

9.4.1   Kaplan-Meier Survival Analysis

Kaplan-Meier survival is NOT an exact measure of survival. Rather, it projects what survival is LIKELY TO BE, if all processes continue on their current path [5]. It has become quite popular in the medical literature, because determining actual 5-year survival requires 5 years FROM THE LAST-ENTERED PATIENT. Projected or actuarial survival is useful because it suggests what survival MIGHT BE in a much shorter period of time and, in addition, it allows for right censoring of patients who are still alive (or lost to follow-up). But the actual survival MIGHT NOT match the actuarial survival and could even be substantially different if the underlying processes change. This was a problem with some early chemotherapy trials in which

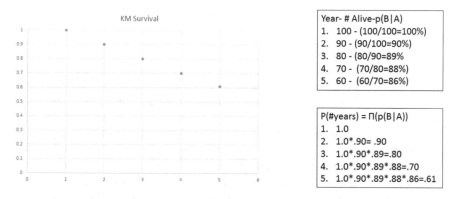

Fig. 9.3 A theoretical Kaplan-Meier survival curve with stepwise calculations

actuarial survival was improved but actual survival was no better. Conceptually, K-M survival is easy to understand. Start entering patients into a study, collecting data based on date of entry (recognizing the possibility of left censoring). As soon as "some" participants surpass the predefined number of years (e.g., actuarial 5-year survival), determine the survival at 1 year after entry for all of the patients ($S1$). Then determine the survival at 2 years, GIVEN the number who were alive at 1 year ($P2$). Calculate this conditional probability of survival for each year, until all patients have been accounted for (keeping in mind right censoring). The actuarial 5-year survival is simply a chain multiplication of conditional probabilities:

$$S(5) = S(1) \times S(2|1) \times S(3|2) \times S(4|3) \times S(5|4)$$

Note, however, that the number of patients contributing the value $S(5|4)$ is often only a small proportion of the total number entered and can be "overweighted" by the earlier periods.

Survival analysis can be accomplished in Excel by "brute force" counting and multiplying. MiniTab has built in functions under the heading (Stat:Reliability/ Survival:DistributionAnalysis) for both right censoring and arbitrary (combinations of left and right) censoring. Once the existence and type of censoring have been established, MiniTab provides options for parametric survival analysis (with choice of 11 distributions) and nonparametric analysis. The Kaplan-Meier approach (Fig. 9.3), based only on proportions in the actual data and not assuming a distribution function, is nonparametric. Once these two options (censoring and distribution) have been addressed, the menu is straightforward. **Kaplan-Meier survival** can be modeled in R using survfit{survival} which also allows censoring as well as staggered enrollment. "survfit" requires defining the outcome variable using a logical statement (status==1 means TRUE for death and status==2 means FALSE for survival). Note specifically the double =, which represents a logical equals rather than a mathematical equals. Both MiniTab and R provide easy options for plotting the survival curve with its corresponding statistics. Additional approaches to survival analysis are found in CRAN:Task View Survival Analysis.

9.4.2 Comparing Survival Curves Using Log-Rank

The **log-rank test** [6] is the most commonly used method for comparing survival between/among groups. In essence, the log-rank test calculates the expected number of deaths at each point where an actual death occurs, and uses the "expected" and "observed" in a variation of the Chi-squared method to evaluate if the curves are not equal. It curiously does not actually involve a log. The log-rank test, also known as the Mantel-Cox test, while fairly robust to non-normality (Chi-squared is nonparametric) does in fact have required assumptions: the relative risk of the outcome remains stable in both groups (proportional hazards) and the survival lines (and the hazards) don't cross. Proportional hazards will be discussed in the next section (Cox proportional hazard analysis). The log-rank test can be accomplished in MiniTab using a specific option within the reliability/survival menu using "right-censored, nonparametric with more than one grouping." The method is straightforward. R accomplishes survival comparison using survdiff{survival}, requiring only the formula and the dataset. $R=0$ defines the traditional log-rank test, but it is also the default.

9.4.3 Evaluating Possible Contributors to Survival

Cox proportional hazards [7], or simply proportional hazards, is an extension of the log-rank test which allows the inclusion of input variables. The test has as its underlying basis the estimation of the hazard function of the combinations of the input variables, but since the baseline hazard appears in each equation, the ratio of equations results in the hazard function cancelling out. Nevertheless, the proportional hazard test has important assumptions [4, 8]: censoring must be non-informative (which means that there isn't a CAUSE of censoring that differs between groups), hazards must actually be proportional (the risk of the event is not influenced by group assignment), and the inputs must be independent and additive (since the input formulation is linear and additive). These assumptions are quite important, as a conclusion drawn when the assumptions are not met is likely to be incorrect. Proportional hazards can be tested, first by looking at a log-log curve of the survival data (which should be a straight line) and then using cox.zph{survival} in R. The actual proportional hazard analysis is accomplished with coxph{survival}. The response variable is a combination of an x-variable (time) and a y-variable (status, usually 0/1) as a "Surv" object. The model formulation is

$$model1 = coxph\left(Surv\left(time, status\right) \sim inputs, data\right)$$

Inputs can be nested, meaning all combinations of each.

The Kaplan-Meier survival curve is very safe. The log-rank has been described as too permissive, and the Cox proportional hazard is often performed without any attention to the assumptions, in situations where the assumptions are limiting—particularly the proportional hazards. K-M and log-rank are relatively safe, but it is essential to test for proportional hazards before performing a Cox analysis.

References

1. Bailar JC, Hoaglin DC. Medical uses of statistics. New York: Wiley; 2012.
2. Bleyer A, Welch HG. Effect of three decades of screening mammography on breast-cancer incidence. N Engl J Med. 2012;367(21):1998–2005.
3. Draisma G, Etzioni R, Tsodikov A, Mariotto A, Wever E, Gulati R, et al. Lead time and overdiagnosis in prostate-specific antigen screening: importance of methods and context. J Natl Cancer Inst. 2009;101:374–83.
4. Bewick V, Cheek L, Ball J. Statistics review 12: survival analysis. Crit Care. 2004;8:389–94.
5. Bland JM, Altman DG. Survival probabilities (the Kaplan-Meier method). BMJ. 1998;317(7172):1572–80.
6. Klein J, Rizzo J, Zhang M, Keiding N. MINI-REVIEW-statistical methods for the analysis and presentation of the results of bone marrow transplants. Part I: unadjusted analysis. Bone Marrow Transplant. 2001;28(10):909–16.
7. Kumar D, Klefsjö B. Proportional hazards model: a review. Reliab Eng Syst Saf. 1994;44(2):177–88.
8. Hess KR. Graphical methods for assessing violations of the proportional hazards assumption in Cox regression. Stat Med. 1995;14(15):1707–23.

Chapter 10
Interpreting Outcomes: Cause and Effect and p-Values

Scenario

A recent article in the New England Journal of Medicine reports the results of a retrospective analysis of factors influencing survival in patients with documented HIV infection. The article concludes that a large number of factors are "statistically significant" and indicates that they are "independent predictors" of outcome. The article concludes by suggesting that efforts to affect these predictors may improve survival. The article is assigned to the monthly infectious disease division journal club. The specific assignment is to determine if the significant input variables are independent, if they are actually predictors, and if it is reasonable to conclude that there is a cause-and-effect relationship.

10.1 The Problem with Assuming Cause and Effect

A large part of the modern medical literature concerns itself with attempts to establish a "cause-effect" relationship: causes of readmission, causes of wound infections, cause of myocardial infarction. It is not widely appreciated that cause and effect CANNOT be established with any confidence using retrospective data from a database. There are many reasons for this, but put most simply, in a retrospective analysis the only options available are the ones that were included in the dataset. These were almost certainly not selected (often many years ago) to answer the question at hand. They are, at best, a convenience sample of all of the variables that COULD have been included. Then, only some of the included variables were actually retained in the analysis. If the study were repeated with a different sample of the same data, would the same variables have been selected? Since there are many other models that COULD have been created, a retrospective study can only SUGGEST what might be. Just because it is "statistically significant" does not mean that it is

© Springer International Publishing Switzerland 2016

P.J. Fabri, *Measurement and Analysis in Transforming Healthcare Delivery*,
DOI 10.1007/978-3-319-40812-5_10

REAL. Only through a prospective, controlled, randomized "experiment" or "trial" can a statement of cause and effect be made. Why is this so? Because only in the PCRT are all of the other factors controlled, leaving only the factor(s) under question to be examined, and then randomizing patients so as to have a "fair" allocation of the factor without bias. And yet, every issue of every medical journal will have articles purporting to establish cause and effect from retrospective data. What CAN be said using a database? At best, a statement of <u>likelihood</u> of a causal relationship, unprovable and untestable.

10.2   Simpson's Paradox and Cause-Effect

Although we have already introduced Simpson's paradox in earlier chapters, it is appropriate at this point, now that we have learned about using outcomes in creating models, to seriously address the issue of cause and effect in its interpretation and application.

The textbook description of Simpson's paradox [1] explains how an outcome can reverse when smaller components are aggregated into larger units. Formal mathematical treatises provide numerous explanations. Underlying these, however, is the fundamental issue, causation. In a prospective, designed experiment, where the factors are actually controlled by the investigator and other factors are minimized by randomization (and subsequently reexamined and verified to be "balanced"), cause and effect can be deduced and subsequently confirmed by repetition. When dealing with retrospectively collected data (which typically were collected for an unrelated purpose), it is tempting to conclude that the included variables are causative and produce the outcome. But there is no actual confirmation of this causative role. In fact, the included variables are often surrogates for other, unmeasured variables with which they are correlated. Often called "lurking" or "hidden" variables, these unmeasured factors are the actual causative factors, yet all we have at hand are the correlated but non-causative variables in the dataset. Said another way, why couldn't the cause be something else that was not actually included in the database? Unfortunately, there is no statistical test or computer method that will sort this out. Since interpretation of an outcome from retrospective data is, by its nature, inferential (inductive rather than deductive), this interpretation is in fact a "conditional probability" (<u>this</u> is the interpretation GIVEN what I know, the data I have, and the inability to infer causation), a likelihood rather than an affirmation. More importantly, it represents only one of a multitude of possible explanations, only one or a few of which were actually tested. The investigator, therefore, must address "how likely" this explanation is, given prior knowledge plus an awareness of the alternatives, which should be thought of as also having "prior probability." The smaller the prior probability, the more strongly the specific outcome needed to "rise to the top." Thus a formal estimate of the likelihood of this outcome versus other plausible explanations should be undertaken. In addition, when a model infers that specific variables are "independent predictors" as is commonly stated in the medical literature, it is important to address both concepts, the "independent" and the "predictor." As mentioned, in a prospective, designed investigation this is straightforward. In a retrospective analysis, it is important to return to the basic analysis of the input variables to revisit their correlation with other inputs as well as correlation with the outcome. In addition, this is an appropriate place for the knowledgeable clinician or investigator to ask the question "does it make sense that this variable could be causative." While formal attribution would require a prospective, designed study, the more plausible the answer, the stronger can be the interpretation.

Bradford-Hill criteria—A more structured approach to this question of causality was proposed and championed by Austin Bradford-Hill, a medical statistician of some note, in 1965 [2–7]. Although his focus was epidemiology, the nine criteria presented by him serve equally well in other domains. The nine criteria will be listed and the interested reader can refer to the bibliography for more in-depth discussion.

A causal relationship should be evaluated by:

1. The strength of the association
2. The consistency of the observed association
3. The specificity of the association
4. The temporal relationship of the association
5. The presence of a biological gradient (dose–response)
6. Biologic plausability
7. Coherence with known facts
8. Presence of experimental or semi-experimental evidence
9. Analogy to other domains

He went on to add "None of my nine viewpoints can bring indisputable evidence for or against the cause and effect hypothesis, and none can be required as a sine qua non."

It would be reasonable to conclude that the more of these supporting principles are present, the more likely a causal relationship exists. It would not be reasonable to conclude that all or most of them should pertain. Nevertheless, a stepwise, formal assessment of these criteria should be performed when inferring a causal relationship from modeling of retrospective data. As further stated by Bradford-Hill, "the required amount of evidence for a causal effect should depend on the possible consequences of interventions derived from causal conclusions."

The frequency of the error of stating causality from retrospective data cannot be overemphasized, nor can the consequences of doing so. Causality should be addressed rigorously and with hesitation. It is sometimes said that the Bradford-Hill criteria are outdated and unnecessarily stringent. This statement must be counterbalanced by a consideration of the consequences of concluding causation when such is not likely.

Similarly, it is important to understand the meaning as well as the misuse of the term "independent." Just as the word probability has two very different meanings (an actual mathematical likelihood versus a statement of "belief"), so too "independent" has two meanings. It could mean that variables are not correlated with each other, or it could mean that the variables serve as inputs (as opposed to the "dependent" output variable(s)). Using the term interchangeably predictably introduces confusion. When "independent" simply means an input variable, it is incorrect to conclude that the variables are independent predictors without actual verification that the variables are truly independent or nearly so.

10.3 p-Values and Types of Error

Our world is surrounded in "p-values": p-Values in the literature, p-values for labo-ratory test rests, p-values in printouts of statistical testing, to name a few. It would be easy to conclude that a p-value says it all. It is frustrating to find an article in which a finding of, say, $p=0.049$ in the experimental group and $p=0.051$ in the control/comparison is interpreted as being different, simply because one is less than 0.05 and ignoring the fact that at two significant figures, they are identical!

Recall that the p-value in hypothesis testing actually indicates not right vs. wrong or good vs. bad, but rather a willingness to be wrong. Also consider the fact that flipping heads four times in a row ($p=0.06$) isn't very uncommon. So the statement that $p<0.05$ actually means that one is willing to be wrong fairly often in saying that the results are repeatable, quite a different statement than the common connotation of "$p<0.05$." Note to self: repeatable?, probably; important?, not necessarily. Conversely, if $p>0.05$ that doesn't mean that the results are NOT repeatable, only that I believe it is less likely to be repeatable.

10.4   Type I and Type II Errors in Hypothesis Testing

Statistical texts describe two types of error in hypothesis testing, type I (α) and type II (β) [8]. Rejecting the null hypothesis ($p<0.05$) and saying that there is a signifi-cant difference, when in truth there is no difference, is known as a type 1 error. This is a conditional probability $P(R|T)$, the probability of <u>rejecting</u> given <u>true</u>, and the 0.05 is the value for alpha. Fortunately, assuming that the sample size is at least 30 (not small), alpha isn't appreciably affected by sample size. This means that the willingness to be wrong when rejecting the null is fairly stable. It also means that increasing sample size doesn't change it appreciably. So once again the key is to first ask the question "is this likely to be true." If current knowledge says that it is not likely (unexpected), then perhaps a smaller value of "p" would be helpful. The current medical literature seems to have a fascination with unexpected findings, without recognizing that something that is unexpected has a low prior probability. This low prior probability changes the posterior conditional probability as well. Even with a very good test (high sensitivity or class conditional probability), an unlikely event is still unlikely. Another consideration must be the consequences of incorrectly rejecting the null hypothesis: the greater the consequence, the more seri-ously should the process be addressed. So when a study rejects the null hypothesis, accepting the alternate hypothesis (commonly defined as $p<0.05$), this result would not likely be different with a larger study and the willingness to be wrong would stay about the same. Therefore the question should be is this a reasonable conclu-sion and can it be applied in a useful way to my patients.

Alternatively, a clinical study may show NO DIFFERENCE ($p>0.05$). A type 2 error is the conditional probability $P(A|F)$ of <u>accepting</u> the null when in fact the null is <u>false</u>, and there actually IS a difference but not shown. This is Beta (β), and $1-\beta$, known as the power of the test, is a measure of how likely a true difference of this magnitude would be identified in a study of this size. Unlike α, the probability of falsely rejecting the null, which is largely independent of sample size, β and its cousin $1 - \beta$ (power) is VERY dependent on sample size. In clinical studies it might require 1000 patients per group to be able to be confident in a statement of no difference. Power of the test can be calculated easily with statistical software, as well as the sample size needed to have a specified level of power. (Minitab has a menu for this (Stat:PowerAndSample Size), and R has a package called {pwr} to accomplish this.) For our purposes, it is important to recognize that the likelihood of a type 2 error, accepting the null when there actually IS a difference, is very dependent on sample size, so small studies that show no difference are questionable whereas very large studies are more convincing but still not conclusive. Whenever a published study concludes NO DIFFERENCE, immediately look in the materials and methods for the analysis of power of the test as well as the sample size that would be needed to confidently say no difference. If nothing is said, it is generally best to ignore such articles. The risk of error is too great. A small study that concludes no difference is not likely to be supported by repeat studies. Larger studies frequently identify the opposite conclusion—that there IS a reason to reject the null hypothesis.

Perhaps a more important issue to consider is whether the result, even if statistically significant, is useful or important. Is increasing survival by a week important CLINICALLY? It may be a major breakthrough in science, leading to future successes, but not be particularly useful in current clinical practice. Answering this question requires advanced subject matter expertise, but should be within the grasp of the treating physician.

10.5   Reinterpreting Sensitivity and Specificity

Every medical student is exposed to the concepts of sensitivity and specificity repeatedly during the course of education and memorizes the definition so as to select it on a multiple choice test. What is little known is that with mandatory external accreditation of clinical laboratories, all laboratory tests have "sufficient" sensitivity and specificity for clinical use (or they wouldn't be offered!). So in today's world, only clinical pathologists have a need to apply sensitivity and specificity to lab tests. Of perhaps more interest is the real meaning of these terms. Let's say that a new lab test is developed for rheumatoid arthritis. In its early testing a large number of individuals with documented, disfiguring RA are brought in and tested. The "sensitivity" is the percentage of individuals with KNOWN rheumatoid arthritis who have a positive test. Commonly, a large number of people who are "known" NOT to have rheumatoid arthritis are also brought in and tested. The specificity is the percentage of individuals who are "known" NOT to have RA who have a negative test. Clearly neither of these represents the actuality in clinical medicine, where the physician is sitting in an office with ONE patient with ONE laboratory result and the actual question, does this patient have RA? Inherent in this question is the fact that the physician must have thought the patient MIGHT have RA before ordering the test (prior probability). But it is less likely that the clinician consciously thought about the actual incidence of RA or the total number of individuals who have a positive test result WHO WERE NOT TESTED (for example, lupus patients). When a clinician is facing a single patient with a single laboratory result, the appropriate question is actually "given a positive laboratory result, what is the likelihood that this patient has RA," or $P(D|+)$. Revisiting Bayes' theorem, this requires knowing the sensitivity PLUS the likelihood of the disease and the overall likelihood of a positive test (all comers). No matter how good the sensitivity of the test, this can't be larger than the likelihood of the disease divided by the total likelihood of a positive test result. With higher incidence/likelihood of disease, this goes up. With more positive test results in individuals with other diseases, this goes down. Consider the Zollinger Ellison syndrome and an elevated serum gastrin level. ZES is extremely rare. Everyone on an H2 blocker or proton pump inhibitor has an elevated gastrin level. So obtaining a gastrin level in a patient with a newly diagnosed but uncomplicated peptic ulcer is overwhelmingly likely to yield an erroneous result. This can be clarified by an understanding of the predicted value of a positive test (the other side of the Bayes' theorem equation). This is in fact the likelihood that the patient with an abnormal laboratory result actually has the disease.

To summarize this discussion on p-values, $p < 0.05$ addresses likely repeatability of a study (confidence). It does not reflect the importance of the study, the usefulness of the result, or the applicability in my practice. $P > 0.05$ on the other hand means that rejecting the null is likely not repeatable, but with an uncertainty that is inversely related to sample size. In clinical use, a result must not only be confident, but it must also be useful and important.

References

1. Tan PN, Steinbach M, Kumar V. Introduction to data mining. Boston: Pearson Addison-Wesley; 2006. p. 384.
2. Winship C, Morgan SL. The estimation of causal effects from observational data. Annu Rev Sociol. 1999;25(1):659–706.
3. Cox DR, Hand DJ, Herzberg AM. Selected statistical papers of Sir David Cox. Cambridge: Cambridge University Press; 2005.
4. Hill AB. The environment and disease: association or causation? 1965. J R Soc Med. 2015;108(1):32–7.
5. Höfler M. The Bradford Hill considerations on causality: a counterfactual perspective. Emerg Themes Epidemiol. 2005;2(1):1.
6. Lucas RM, McMichael AJ. Association or causation: evaluating links between "environment and disease". Bull World Health Organ. 2005;83(10):792–5.
7. Morgan SL, Winship C. Counterfactuals and causal inference: methods and principles for social research, vol. xiii. New York: Cambridge University Press; 2007. 319 p.
8. Crawley MJ. Statistics an introduction using R. 2nd ed. Hoboken: Wiley; 2014.

Chapter 11
Useful Tools

Scenario
Dr. Sally Worth is a neuroradiologist at a preeminent neurosurgical institute, which has just installed an intraoperative MRI and is preparing to "launch" it. The hospital COO has convened a group of "knowledge experts" to conduct a failure mode and effect analysis prior to authorizing the electrical connections to the device. Sally is asked to gather the information from the nominal group process into a structured Excel spreadsheet, set up to facilitate a modified two-step Delphi process to identify the most likely things that can go wrong as well as their frequency, severity, and undetectability. She is also instructed to identify tiers of importance based on the number of standard deviations. Finally, she is asked to set up an np-type statistical process control chart to track the occurrence of the most likely failure mode over time.

11.1 Tools for Understanding and Applying Analytical Methods

While there are many useful tools for understanding and applying analytical methods, three are particularly important for the clinician interested in analytics: outlier and anomaly detection, statistical process control (SPC), and failure mode and effect analysis (FMEA).

11.2 Outlier/Anomaly Detection

What in fact does an "abnormal lab test" mean? Analysis of how the clinical pathologists establish the normal ranges (mean ± 2SD from a presumably "healthy" population) would indicate that 2.5 % of all healthy patients will have an abnormal

© Springer International Publishing Switzerland 2016
P.J. Fabri, *Measurement and Analysis in Transforming Healthcare Delivery*,
DOI 10.1007/978-3-319-40812-5_11

low result and 2.5 % an abnormal high result. (If the result is not normally distributed but skewed to higher values, it would actually be higher than 2.5 %.) Taking this a step further, if we do a panel of 20 laboratory tests, using the same definition of "abnormal," 2 out of every 3 healthy patients would be expected to have at least one abnormal laboratory result $(1-(1-0.05)^{20})$. These are called "outliers." Hawkins defines an outlier as "an observation that differs so much from other observations as to arouse suspicion that it was generated by a different mechanism" [1]. The analytical methods described in this text are all intended to identify patterns or predictability in a dataset. They "improve" if outliers are eliminated. There are situations, however, in which identifying deviation from patterns, or **anomalies**, is the goal. As noted by Taleb [2], outliers are often viewed as nuisances to be removed; yet sometimes outliers are even more interesting than the rest of the data. In either case, to identify and remove outliers or to recognize and study them, a structured approach to identifying and verifying outlier status is essential. Aggarwal [3] presents a comprehensive analysis of a very large number of methods for outlier/anomaly detection. We will limit our discussion to a few relevant methods.

The very concept of an outlier or anomaly requires first a definition of outlier FROM WHAT. Outlier status is then based on some statement of HOW DIFFERENT from the expected is required to be able to say something is unexpected, which requires some measurement of distance from as opposed to stochastic variation (random variability) which is simultaneously occurring. In other words, an outlier must be so far away from what is expected HERE that it must belong someplace else. This is certainly starting to sound a lot like statistics, which in fact it is. Just refocused. Outlier detection applies almost all of the concepts in all the previous chapters to the new question at hand—is this an outlier. Put another way, being an outlier essentially means that if I used a statistical test with the assumption of being wrong once in 20, then this is one of those times. While the term "error" is often applied to this situation, it isn't an error in the sense of "a mistake." Rather, it's "just one of those things" that happens.

As was seen earlier, distance from can be thought of at least three different ways: distance from a model (such as a normal distribution), distance greater than a predefined amount, and difference in density. In addition, there can be more than one variable and thus more than one distance. How many of these distances are meaningful? Important?

In a model-based approach, the actual distribution of "from" must first be established using techniques now familiar, keeping in mind that many variables follow distributions quite different from normal (such as measures of time, failure, or lab tests based on an exponential relationship like light absorption or enzyme kinetics).

Assuming a suitable distribution can be identified, a univariate approach looks remarkably like a t-test, with a predefined number of standard deviations (recall that standard deviations apply to individual measurements, while standard errors apply to means—an outlier is an individual measurement) for outlier status. Thus if the distance of a value is more than, say, 2 SD, and is only considered an outlier in one direction, a one-tailed t-test (or z-test) would say that the value has a 95 % likelihood of being an outlier. For 3 SD, 99 %. This can be accomplished in R, using Grubb's test (grubbs.test{outliers}). Three different forms of Grubb's test are available (known as types 10, 11, and 20), and all three should be run in that sequence. Type 10 will identify a single outlier on one or the other side of a normal distribution (the data can obviously be transformed prior to running the test for other distributions); type 11 attempts to identify one outlier on each side; and type 20 tries to find 2 outliers on one or the other side. Comparing the results of the three runs provides an overview of the outlier status.

In a multivariate approach, we can revisit the Mahalanobis distance [1], a distance away in multidimensional, standardized space. This is a common approach to defining an outlier:

$$\text{Mahalanobis}\left(x, \bar{x}\right) = \left(\left(x - \bar{x}\right) S^{-1} \left(x - \bar{x}\right)^{T}\right.$$

which on close inspection is actually the multivariate formulation of the distance squared divided by the standard deviation.

In MiniTab, outlier visualization can be obtained using (Stat:Multivariate:Princi palComponent:Graphs:OutlierPlot). The resulting graph highlights outliers above the line (the value for a point can be identified by rolling over it with the cursor). In R, numerous advanced applications of Mahalanobis distance are provided in package {mvoutlier}.

A similar approach can be used with any analytical method that provides an "expected" result. An outlier is simply a result that was not "expected," typically based on a measure of 2 SD from the central tendency or a residual greater than 2 SD.

11.3 Statistical Process Control

During the early years of industrial advancement, products, such as automobiles, were manufactured one at a time. Early efforts at increasing productivity are attributed to Frederick Taylor and his approach to manufacturing known as Taylorism [4]. Taylor measured how long it took workers to accomplish individual tasks and then assigned individuals to do repetitive tasks. Products were simple then and application of these principles appeared to improve productivity. Henry Ford took this concept and added the assembly line—the product-in-process moved past the workers who were doing repetitive tasks [5]. It soon became apparent that doing repetitive tasks could be boring and lead to error. Inspectors were added to the end of the assembly line and defective product was identified and "reworked." But soon products became too complex for reliable terminal inspection, leading to defective products known as "lemons." Consider modern medicine, having originated in the "art" of treating one patient at a time, with a perception of individual attention and high quality but evolving into high volume, procedurally dominated treatment (e.g., hernia repair hospitals, free-standing MRI units, or parathyroidectomy surgicenters!) What was once simple has become complex and repetitive, but without "inspectors."

Walter Shewhart was an engineer at a division of Bell Laboratories known as the Western Electric Company. Shewhart introduced a mathematical/graphic methodology which he named statistical process control (SPC) for assessing variability in product metrics that could actually be used by manufacturing workers on the shop floor. This graphical approach, demonstrating "control limits" in standard deviations, utilizes two different methodologies: evaluating attributes (defective vs. not defective) and measuring variables (measurements) [6]. Attribute charts can monitor either the number of units that have some number of defects (defectives) or the actual number of defects. Two types of attribute charts were developed for **defectives**, the p-chart which tracked the proportion of defective products (consider the percent readmissions after hospital discharge) and the np-chart which tracked the number of defective products (number of UTIs per month). Charts were also developed for **defects** per unit sampled (u-charts and c-charts), which addressed more than one defect per defective product (number of complications during a hospital stay).

Charts looking specifically at measured values (variable charts) were based on measures of central tendency (mean or median) and variability (range or standard deviation) such as daily values for a glucose control sample in a hospital laboratory. In each of these specific types of charts, the horizontal axis is unit number, date, or time, depicting the course of a continuous process, and a vertical axis measured in units of variability, often the fractional number of standard deviations (±3 SD, or 99 % tolerance, is usually taken as a the measure of "out of control"). The central tendency and the variability are usually estimated from an initial pilot study or from historical data. The dimensions of the SPC axes are constructed from these pilot measures, and data points are entered at regular sampling intervals (which could be every unit, every shift, every day, etc.). Clinical situations where SPC could be useful include monthly wound infection rates, hospital readmission rates, door-to-balloon times in cardiac catheterization, etc. Shewhart's important contribution was to make variation large enough to cause concern easily visible. This was accomplished by quantifying the number of standard deviations and clearly marking plus and minus 1, 2, and 3 standard deviations. A set of "rules," known as the Western Electric rules [7], established when a process was "out of control," requiring specific attention, distinguishing this from normal random variability. Random variability he called "controlled" and additional variability "uncontrolled," comparable to the statistical concepts of general variance and special variance. A single observation beyond 3 SD from the mean is equivalent to $p < 0.01$ and was reason to "stop the line." 2 out of 3 consecutive points beyond 2 SD, 4 out of 5 consecutive points beyond 1 SD, or 8 consecutive points all above or all below the mean each have the same meaning.

In clinical practice, after identifying some measurable component (attribute or variable) that is important, definition of attribute versus variable and an initial assessment of mean and standard deviation allow creation of the appropriate SPC chart. This can be accomplished in Excel by manually creating a scatterplot graph or in Minitab under "Stat:ControlCharts." Minitab is designed to apply the Western Electric rules to identify when the process needs careful assessment. The three most useful SPC charts for clinical use are the p-chart, np-chart, and Xbar-SD chart. The p-chart, used for tracking the proportion of defectives, can be created in Minitab using (Stat:ControlCharts:AttributesChart:p). The parameters for the control limits can be set in "p-Options." The p-chart would be useful for tracking wound infection rates, readmission rates, etc. as a fraction of the full population at risk. The np-chart tracks the <u>number</u> of events (counts) as in number of residents with duty hour violations per month or the number of DVTs in a monthly sample of 20 asymptomatic patients. For quantitative measurement data, such as monthly dollar expenditure for the operating room disposable supplies, a variable Xbar-S (mean and SD) chart would identify a change in usage patterns (Stat:ControlChart:VariableChart Subgroups:Xbar-S). The powerful advantage of control charts is that, once set up, an individual without statistical experience can track an activity and visually identify if there is a notable change. In particular, SPC is a useful tool for the continuous evaluation of "before and after" data, where the before data are used to create the mean (normal) or median (non-normal) and the control limits, and the after data are entered as they are measured, allowing an early identification of a change when a Western Electric rule demonstrates one.

11.4 Failure Mode and Effect Analysis

Similarly grounded in manufacturing, the FMEA [8] allows "**brainstorming**" when a new process or piece of equipment is ready to be started. By bringing together a group of knowledgeable individuals, under the protection of a safe, structured brainstorming process, a comprehensive list of "what could go wrong" (failure modes) is generated. A common technique for this brainstorming process is the **nominal group process (NGP)** [9]. The NGP provides the structure and control necessary to make the activity "safe" for all participants, even the shy ones. Once a comprehensive list is identified, prioritization can then be accomplished using a modified Delphi process [10] (two or more iterative surveys which score each failure mode), which identifies the consensus opinion. Repetition of the survey, including the average results of the prior iteration, tends to develop convergence, which is interpreted as consensus. The prioritized list can then be used to implement a strategy to minimize risk.

An FMEA is an appropriate approach when a new system, process, or piece of equipment has been selected, has been identified as having risk, and is about to be put into use. Any type of risk would be appropriate, but safety of use, operational failure, and hazardous exposure are common in medicine. If there is no perceived risk (buying new waiting room chairs), an FMEA would probably be "overkill."

Selecting the FMEA team is important. At least five and probably no more than ten members seems to work best, although for a very complex situation more diverse input may be required. Group dynamics seem to change with more than ten participants. Individuals whose knowledge and expertise span the entire risk domain should be included. Since some individuals might be reluctant to identify "unpopular" failure modes, or would be uncomfortable in a hierarchical environment, it is important to understand the dynamics of the group prior to meeting. Typically a single meeting is sufficient, but subsequent "homework" is required.

A strong leader of the process is essential, who is firmly grounded in the method of the nominal group process. The success of the NGP depends largely on the ability of the leader to maintain control over the process without inhibiting creativity while simultaneously "protecting" the shyer members.

The two most important considerations are "what is the question" and making the process "safe" for all participants. "What is the question" actually requires some thought, as the output of the NGP depends completely on the appropriateness and clarity of the question. "What could go wrong when the intraoperative MRI is used" would be an appropriate question. "How can we improve safety in the OR" would be unlikely to identify failure modes when an intraoperative MRI suite is activated. Making the process safe is critical, as once someone becomes uncomfortable with the process it will probably fail or at least be limited in scope.

It is helpful to have a whiteboard or posterboard with the question clearly printed so that all can see it. It is also helpful to have a dedicated "scribe," to enter the identified items into a projected spreadsheet column exactly as stated. The leader provides a brief introduction to the problem and identifies the question, reminding the group to focus on the question. This will limit unintended "hidden agendas." If a member strays from the question, it is easy (and non-threatening) to just point to the question on the whiteboard. The leader then explains that the process will "go around the room," specifying the direction, and that anyone can "pass" on any given round without forfeiting subsequent rounds. The process continues going around the group until nobody has anything additional to add. The leader should explain at the beginning that there will be no comments or discussion of any suggestion, nor will any suggestion be deleted or modified. If a suggestion is poorly stated or confusing, the leader should simply state "please clarify." Although the scribe can shorten a suggestion to a few words, it is important that the exact suggestion is written down. Sometimes the most timid person in the room has the critical suggestion. Clearly the role of the leader in this process is important.

Once there are no more suggestions from the group, the leader should ask the group if anyone sees duplicates or doesn't understand any of the suggestions. At this point, the safety of the group members is no longer critical. The leader should then explain next steps. The NGP is typically followed by a modified Delphi process, which is easily conducted remotely. The leader should explain that an Excel spreadsheet with an alphabetical list (to completely remove any memory of "order" or "who" during the initial meeting) of the identified failure modes will be sent out to each member. To the right of each failure mode will be columns for scoring three characteristics of each failure mode (effects): frequency, severity, and undetectability. The leader should clearly explain (and the spreadsheet should contain explicit instructions) that this is NOT RANKING. Each failure mode should be scored, based on the individual's experience, using the appropriate scale. Typical publications on the scoring process describe a ten-point scale, with 1 being low and 10 high. A 5-point scale, however, is simpler and seems to work well with physicians. The leader should explain that 1 means extremely unlikely, 5 very likely, 3 average with 2 and 4 filling in between. The leader should also explain that "undetectability" is a backwards scale, with 5 being VERY UNDETECTABLE. The leader should then set the timeline for returning the received spreadsheets, which should be short, and clarify that the spreadsheet will be sent two times. The second time, the average results from the first iteration will be visibly included in the spreadsheet. Seeing the "average response" is the mechanism of converging opinion, yet allowing individuals with strong opinions to persist in the second iteration.

After the meeting, the leader should edit the list of failure modes, assuring that each is clear and concise without changing the meaning, and then alphabetize the list, thus eliminating the "sequence" effect that occurred during the meeting. Having then received the returned spreadsheets from the first iteration, the leader should determine the average and the standard deviation for each component of each failure mode and enter these in new columns added to the spreadsheet. The averages of the first iteration will be sent to the members, whereas the standard deviations will be kept by the leader. The second iteration should thus be the same spreadsheet but with three new columns (the first round means for frequency, severity, and undetectability) added, each followed to the right by a blank column for the second scoring. The instructions should be included again in the second iteration, once more reminding participants that this is SCORING, NOT RANKING. The leader should then analyze the second iteration, just as the first. Convergence of opinion is verified by a narrowing in the standard deviation, with the second average reflecting a more advanced group opinion than the first. The Delphi process is not necessarily limited to two iterations, but it seems possible to get physicians to complete two rounds, if they are told in advance. The leader should then determine the overall average and standard deviation for the average scores of the second iteration. Lack of agreement on a particular failure mode is identified by a standard deviation higher than the overall standard deviation. Finally, the leader should calculate the "risk priority number (RPN)" for each failure mode by multiplying the scores for frequency, severity, and undetectability in a spreadsheet column to the right. With all the individual RPNs calculated, calculate the average and SD of the RPN and sort the spreadsheet based on the RPN, placing a line at the overall average, the overall average +1 and +2 standard deviations. Failure modes above $\bar{x} + 2SD$ (the high outliers) should be addressed immediately, and then the list continued as long as time and resources permit.

11.4.1   Summary

The intent of this presentation of statistical methods to improve healthcare delivery is to provide clinicians and clinical investigators with an up-to-date and rigorous approach to the analysis of data. This approach is based on the well-established engineering concept that in order to improve something it has to be measured. In the case of healthcare, this means outcomes. But outcomes data typically are "mined" from databases that were collected for other purposes, by other people, and are thus often mired in error and misunderstanding. In addition, the development of powerful desktop computers has allowed the development of newer and more sophisticated analytical methods that were specifically designed to address the limiting assumptions of the earlier, "traditional" analytical methods. As the proverb says "It is better to light one candle than to curse the darkness."

The analytical approach used throughout this text uses Microsoft Excel as "home" for all data analysis, performs initial descriptive analysis and graphic visualization in Excel, and then "pushes" the data into more powerful analytical software, notably menu-driven MiniTab and the more difficult but extremely sophisticated "R." Since "R" requires writing often complex and syntactically demanding code, the middle-ware "RExcel" or "Rcmdr" provides a menu-driven approach for many of the advanced methods and, at the least, a starting point for additional methods.

Inherent in these discussions is the principle that all retrospective analysis is in fact inferential, rather than deductive, so a clear and accurate understanding of the data, the assumptions, and the limitations is essential to proper interpretation.

Within each analytical domain, methods are presented starting with the most traditional followed by more modern and advanced approaches, usually describing approaches in both MiniTab and "R." It is my belief that these concepts are well within the understanding of a reasonably well-prepared and motivated physician who is committed to continuous, life-long learning and knows how to use a search engine. Most questions can be answered by a search using the desired term plus Excel, Minitab, or CRAN.

References

1. Tan PN, Steinbach M, Kumar V. Introduction to data mining. Boston: Pearson-Addison Wesley; 2006. 769 p.
2. Taleb N. The black swan: the impact of the highly improbable. 1st ed. New York: Random House; 2007.
3. Aggarwal CC. Outlier analysis. New York: Springer; 2013.
4. Littler CR. Understanding taylorism. Br J Sociol. 1978;29:185–202.
5. Doray B, Macey D. From taylorism to fordism: a rational madness. London: Free Association Books; 1988.
6. Benneyan J, Lloyd R, Plsek P. Statistical process control as a tool for research and healthcare improvement. Qual Saf Health Care. 2003;12(6):458–64.
7. Klein M. Two alternatives to the Shewhart X control chart. J Qual Technol. 2000;32(4):427.
8. McDermott RE, Mikulak RJ, Beauregard MR. The basics of FMEA. 2nd ed. New York: Productivity Press; 2009.
9. Delbecq AL, Van de Ven AH. A group process model for problem identification and program planning. J Appl Behav Sci. 1971;7(4):466–92.
10. Hsu CC, Sandford BA. The Delphi technique: making sense of consensus. Pract Assess Res Eval. 2007;12(10):1–8.

Appendix
Using R

Appendix A: A Few Basic Rules

As discussed early in this volume, "R" can be a very frustrating software package, but the "price" is more than justified by its relevance and power. The easiest way to make "R" user friendly is to use RExcel or RCommander as middleware, which provides easy transferability between R and Excel, drop-down menus for the commonly used statistical tests, linear models, and graphics. But the more advanced methods require writing R-code, which is case sensitive and absolutely unforgiving. This brief description of R is intended to address a number of specific problems typically faced when using R and is not intended as a comprehensive introduction or manual of R, since numerous such materials are readily available, often electronically. "The R Book" by Michael Crawley provides a comprehensive discussion of the R language in Chap. 1, and "Statistics: An Introduction Using R" by Crawley or "Introductory Statistics with R" by Dalgaard explain all the major statistical methods using "R."

Let me repeat—R is absolutely case sensitive. If a variable name is misspelled or even if one letter is in the wrong case, R will reply that the variable does not exist, without any help or suggestions that there is a problem. Since most of the advanced methods are based on or similar to the simpler or more common methods, it is often helpful to use RExcel to write a "prototype" of the more common method and then make the necessary modifications to the code. Whenever possible, use one of the "R" drop-down lists to select files or variables to avoid having to type them. One way or another, writing code is unavoidable, but literally following instructions minimizes the errors.

Where are the instructions? The "overseers" of R require that all methods in all packages MUST follow a set of syntax rules, be accompanied by instructions in a very standardized and explicit format, and include working examples. It is tempting to skip the help in the belief that errors won't occur, but literally following the rules is the best way to avoid mistakes. Detailed and specific instructions can be found with a Google search using the term "CRAN" plus the name of the method.

© Springer International Publishing Switzerland 2016
P.J. Fabri, *Measurement and Analysis in Transforming Healthcare Delivery*,
DOI 10.1007/978-3-319-40812-5

How are mistakes in "R" identified? Unlike other software, that provides an audible or visible clue that an error has occurred, R simply moves to the next line, the only evidence being the absence of an answer. The only way to know if a method worked is to ask for the output. This is simplified by following a standardized approach to writing code:

1. Always read the instructions and follow them literally.
2. Name your variables (either in Excel prior to transfer or renaming in "R") wisely, using only lower case, simple names, and no symbols.
3. Provide a name for each method. After "running" a model, type in the method name to see the output.
4. Use simple names for models (model1, model2, etc.). While it might seem appropriate to provide meaningful names, that just means more typing errors, particularly when compound names or capital letters are used.
5. R uses right arrows to link the assignment name to the equation, but these can be replaced with equal (=) without harm. R does this because "equal" already has a meaning in R and "exactly equal," $\equiv$, an even narrower one. Note that in name assignment, an equal sign does NOT mean mathematical equality, but only logical equality, mapping what is on the right to the name on the left. Telling R that something actually equals some value requires a 3-bar equal sign ($\equiv$), exactly equal.
6. The simple name on the left side followed by an equal sign maps (and names) the output of whatever is accomplished on the right side. This means that the entire right side can be called up by typing the name from the left side.
7. After the method has been run, simply typing the name for the model (e.g., "model1") will produce the output. Adding $ and an attribute after the model name will provide the specific result of the attribute.

Where is HELP for writing code located? First, enter "CRAN" in a search engine followed by a term that describes the method you are seeking (e.g., CRAN linear regression). The first two or three items displayed will be the contents of a package, the formal syntax, and usually a review article that describes the underlying logic/math/science. Examine all of them and save them in a folder of R methods—so that you can find them easily next time!

Appendix B: Interpreting the Documentation

Each package has a name (which similarly must be entered EXACTLY) and contains a variable number of interrelated methods and usually a few relevant datasets. Within the package contents is a succinct explanation of the method and the syntax, but it is rarely "enough." Examining the page of syntax (**R documentation**) provides all of the necessary information. Each R-documentation report is laid out in exactly the same way:

- The R **name** for the method followed in curly brackets by the package name (each will be used); the full "title" of the method; a brief **description** of the purpose of the method.

- **"Usage,"** which contains the exact syntax for writing the code and the order that R expects to see them.
- **"Arguments"** contains the input variables, many of which have defaults.
- **"Value"** includes the list of outputs of the method.
- **"References"** includes two or three relevant but "dense" articles.
- **"See Also"** includes hyperlinks to related methods.
- **"Examples"** contains the R-code to run an example, so it can be copied into the RConsole and run.

A better way is to enter example(method name) into R and it will run the example. In addition, R frequently has additional outputs which are not shown until asked for. This is accomplished by appending $ followed by "attributes" after the name of the method (method$attributes). A listing of available attributes is displayed. Then typing the method name, $, and the attribute name will provide the output for the attribute.

Appendix C: Linear Regression

Linear regression is one of the fundamental underpinnings of advanced analytics and will serve as a useful example of R code and syntax. The method for fitting a linear model in "R" is named "lm" and is located in the package **"stats" (lm{stats})**. This can be found most easily by doing a search for "CRAN lm" or "CRAN linear regression" and clicking "R:Fitting Linear Models." A standard-format **R Documentation** appears, beginning with lm{stats}, indicating that the notation to invoke the method is **lm**, contained in the package **stats**. As always, it begins with a very brief statement of what the method accomplishes.

Usage provides the actual coding syntax for the method (sometimes with more than one version, but the first one listed matches the most recent version of R):

lm(formula, data, subset, weights, na.action, method="qr", model=TRUE, x=FALSE, y=FALSE, qr=TRUE, singular.ok=TRUE, contrasts=NULL, offset,...)

The description of each term can be found under Arguments. The most important (and the only required term) is "formula." For "R," formula means an expression **y ~ x**, in which "y" is the output and "x" is the input set of variables in column form. But "R" needs to know where the data are coming from. While it might seem logical that R would know, IT DOESN'T, so it has to be told and regularly by simply including the exact name of the dataset. Alternatively, a command "attach()" creates a strong link between R and a dataset, but that very tight connection will have to be undone with "unattach." In other words, if a dataset is attached to "R," R will search ONLY in the named dataset to find all of the variables in $y \sim x$. It is generally safer to specify the dataset in each method UNLESS you don't plan to use any other datasets or subsets. Since it is often useful to make subsets of the original dataset in the model of a project, forgetting to unattach and then attach means that you will likely end up using the wrong data. "R" won't know and neither will you. This is a particular risk because of a very useful expression $y\sim$. (y-tilde followed by a period). $y\sim$. creates a model using y as the output and ALL OTHER VARIABLES in the named or attached dataframe as the input variable. Specific columns can be defined either be deleting or by adding: the command [-3] uses all of the variables EXCEPT the third column; or alternatively typing each of the included variable names separated by + signs will include each named variable. So if you had an original dataset named "readmission" but later deleted a number of columns and named that readmission2, attaching "readmission" would mean that R would consistently use the original dataset. So at a minimum, the code for a linear model would be $lm(y\sim x,data)$. "**Details**" provides a succinct but useful description of the method and "**Value**" describes all of the results included in the default output. Note that in this method both the Arguments and Value are described as "object of class lm." R is an "object-oriented" programming language, which means that it operates on "chunks," referred to as objects. An object is most easily thought of as anything that can be cut and pasted. Formally, an **object** is an **entity** that has **properties** and **actions**. Properties are characteristics that can be set, like "bold." Actions tell the operating system to actually DO SOMETHING. As an example, "Delete" is an action, which is understood by the operating system, so typing or clicking on delete accomplishes a specified action. A word, a number, a shape, or an entire Beatles song can be handled as an object. But that object belongs to a named class and has a predefined format that includes a set of available properties and actions. In R, equations, methods, models, etc. are all stored as objects, so knowing the properties of a class of objects and the attributes that that class generates tells all that is necessary.

Under **Value** additional information is provided: the commands **summary()** and **anova()** are generic functions that can be found associated with most analytic methods. **Summary** provides a succinct summary of the output and **anova** produces the analysis of variance. Following is a list of outputs provided by **lm**. In this case, the outputs listed are the same as the **attributes** of the model, but on occasion, **attributes** produces additional information. Also within **value** is a statement about **time series**, another method for looking at serial data but with equal intervals of time represented as x.

Continuing in the R Document, after **Authors** and **References**, R provides links to related topics worth examining in **See Also**. Finally, R provides an example. Copying and pasting the example, exactly as written, into the RConsole (native R) or RCommander (RExcel) will tell R to execute the example, typically including all of the available output and graphs. The same information can be obtained by entering example(lm) into the console.

Since all of the R documentation follows this format and structure, understanding this approach to the documentation should make using a new method straightforward. To repeat, if a method in R doesn't work, it is usually because the instructions in the R documentation were not followed EXACTLY or case sensitivity was violated.

Appendix D: Selecting and Installing a Package

Often a search of a method name will provide more than one package that contains a variation of the requested method. Recall that packages in R are written by actual expert users, who typically wrote a package using R for a specific purpose and then submitted it to CRAN for potential "publication." Often more than one investigator develops a package, typically for specific applications of the method, that contains the desired method, but with differing syntax, specifications, or outputs. Often (but not always!) earlier packages are more basic and subsequent packages have more "accessories" or "options." Numerous packages contain methods to accomplish linear regression, so it may be helpful to exam the R documentation for each and choose the version that best fits the application.

Installing a package in R can be a frustrating experience as well, but by following a few simple rules, it can usually be accomplished. Once a needed package has been identified, the easiest way to install it is to use the native RConsole. In the top menu, select **Packages**, followed by **Install Package.** In a few seconds, a pop-up named **CRAN mirror** will appear. Pick any location, although it may be preferable to select one that is geographically close (for example, USA(TX1). Another pop-up will subsequently show an alphabetical list of all of the available packages. Note that this list is being updated and renewed on a regular basis. Additional information on a specific R package can be found by searching "**available CRAN packages by name.**" A listing of newly contributed packages (by date range) is available by searching "**R what's new.**" A number of useful tools can be found under "Help" in RConsole:Manuals (An Introduction to R, R Reference, R Data Import/Export, FAQ on R, etc.)

After installing a package, it resides in your hard drive. But that does NOT mean that R knows this! When either RConsole or RExcel with RCommander is opened, the R environment underlying the visual interface is essentially a blank slate, with a few designated packages automatically opened. However, each time you open "R," whether through RConsole or RCommander you need to load (not reinstall, they're there!) any other needed packages. This is accomplished by entering "library(package)" or alternatively, in RExcel, Tools:LoadPackage (once a package has been installed, it will appear in the LoadPackage menu). If the project requires several packages, load all of them, allowing use of ALL of the methods. Once a package is loaded, "library(help=package)" displays the contents of the package, allowing confirmation of spelling/case of the methods. "help(method)" provides the R documentation for the method. One of the peculiarities of R is that once a package has been <u>installed,</u> it can be accessed either by RConsole RCommander. But <u>loading</u> the package is specific to the console being used. Even if both RConsole and RCommander are opened, they do not talk to each other. RConsole is simple to operate but requires writing code. Hitting "enter" submits the code. RCommander is a menu-driven way to write the code. RCommander requires clicking on SUBMIT. Hitting "enter" in RCommander simply does a carriage return/line feed and doesn't run the code. You will receive no warning or alarm. The only way to know that nothing happened is the absence of an output.

Appendix E: Another Summary for Actually Using R

First, clean up the dataset in Excel and "put" it into RExcel using a right click followed by "R" and "Put Data." Or import it into RCommander using the import Excel spreadsheet command in RCommander. Identify what method you want to use. If the method is already contained in the menus of RExcel, proceed with the menu and use the help function and the pop-ups. For new methods, perform a search using "CRAN" and the name of the method. On the top left corner of the R-documentation, the case-sensitive term for the method as well as the package are specified. Using RConsole, install the package and then switch to RExcel or RCommander to load the package using "library(package)." Most methods only require specifying the formula, the dataset, and one or two inputs, leaving the remainder as defaults. Write the code for the model by first giving it a name (e.g., model1), then equals, and then the syntax, being careful to use the exact case and spelling as well as order of terms. After submitting the code, identify the available output options by entering model1$attributes or attributes(model1). Most of these will also be listed under Value in the R-documentation. Pay particular attention to the available function that measures how well the model performs (R-squared, mean squared error, AIC, BIC, etc.). Continue running additional methods that suit the purpose, comparing and selecting the method that works best.

Task	Links for "R-Methods"	Package name	Link
Classification	Neural network	neuralnet, nnet	https://cran.r-project.org/web/packages/NeuralNetTools/index.html
Clustering	Partitioning	cluster	https://cran.r-project.org/web/packages/cluster/cluster.pdf
Clustering	Rpart/party (conditional inference tree)/ mvpart	rpart	https://cran.r-project.org/web/packages/rpart/rpart.pdf
Classification	Random forests randomForest	rpart	https://cran.r-project.org/web/packages/rpart/rpart.pdf
Classification	Bundling/bagging/ ensemble ipred	rpart	https://cran.r-project.org/web/packages/rpart/rpart.pdf
Regression	Shrinkage lasso/ lasso2/lars	lars	https://cran.r-project.org/web/packages/lars/lars.pdf
Classification/ regression	Penalized LDA	penalizedLDA	https://cran.r-project.org/web/packages/penalizedLDA/penalizedLDA.pdf
Classification	Pamr shrunken centroids classifier	pamr	https://cran.r-project.org/web/packages/pamr/pamr.pdf
Classification	Boosting gbm	gbm	https://cran.r-project.org/web/packages/gbm/gbm.pdf
Classification/ regression	SVM/e1071/kernlab/	e1071	https://cran.r-project.org/web/packages/e1071/e1071.pdf

Task	Links for "R-Methods"	Package name	Link
Association analysis	Arules apriori eclat	arules	https://cran.r-project.org/web/packages/arules/arules.pdf
Classification	Fuzzy frbs	frbs	https://cran.r-project.org/web/packages/frbs/frbs.pdf
Support vector machines	Tune e1071	e1071	https://cran.r-project.org/web/packages/e1071/e1071.pdf
	Svmpath for C	svmpath	https://cran.r-project.org/web/packages/svmpath/svmpath.pdf
Evaluation	ROCR	ROCR	https://cran.r-project.org/web/packages/ROCR/index.html
Classification/ regression	Caret	caret	https://cran.r-project.org/web/packages/caret/caret.pdf
Regression/ classification	Partial least squares-PLSDA	misOmics	https://cran.r-project.org/web/packages/mixOmics/mixOmics.pdf
Regression	Multiple regression	MASS (lm)	http://www.statmethods.net/stats/regression.html
Regression	Best subset regression	bestglm	https://cran.r-project.org/web/packages/bestglm/vignettes/bestglm.pdf
Classification	Hierarchical classification	cluster	https://cran.r-project.org/web/views/Cluster.html
Classification	Logistic regression (use logit link)	MASS	http://www.r-bloggers.com/how-to-perform-a-logistic-regression-in-r/
Clustering	Hierarchical clustering	stats(glm)	https://stat.ethz.ch/R-manual/R-devel/library/stats/html/hclust.html
Outlier analysis	Outlier analysis	outliers	https://cran.r-project.org/web/packages/outliers/outliers.pdf
Understanding/ visualization	Descriptive statistics		http://rtutorialseries.blogspot.com/2009/11/r-tutorial-series-summary-and.html
Understanding/ visualization	Plot		http://www.r-bloggers.com/how-to-plot-a-graph-in-r/
Understanding/ visualization	Histogram		https://stat.ethz.ch/R-manual/R-devel/library/graphics/html/hist.html
Statistics	ANOVA	stats	http://www.statmethods.net/stats/anova.html
Survival	Survival	survival	https://cran.r-project.org/web/views/Survival.html
Survival	Cox regression	survival	https://stat.ethz.ch/R-manual/R-devel/library/survival/html/coxph.html
Regression/ classification	lars	lars	https://cran.r-project.org/web/packages/lars/lars.pdf
Regression/ classification	Lasso	lars	https://cran.r-project.org/web/packages/lars/lars.pdf

Task	Links for "R-Methods"	Package name	Link
Regression/ classification	Principal component regression	pls	https://cran.r-project.org/web/ packages/pls/pls.pdf
Regression/ classification	Ridge regression	MASS	https://stat.ethz. ch/R-manual/R-devel/library/ MASS/html/lm.ridge.html
Regression/ classification	Partial least square regression	pls	https://cran.r-project.org/web/ packages/pls/pls.pdf
Classification	Bayesian belief network	bnlearn	https://cran.r-project.org/web/ packages/bnlearn/bnlearn.pdf
Classification	Naïve Bayes analysis	e1071	https://cran.r-project.org/web/ packages/e1071/e1071.pdf
Understanding/ visualization	Table		https://stat.ethz.ch/R-manual/ R-devel/library/base/html/table. html

Glossary

ANOVA two-factor with replication* ANOVA with two major "categories" or factors, typically with more than two groups (columns) and two or more subsets (sets of rows with multiple entries in each).

ANOVA without replication* An ANOVA method for pseudo-replication which reduces multiple measurements of the same data point to the average of the measures.

Array An ordered set of data with two or more "dimensions." A two-dimensional array is called a matrix.

Array Function* In Excel, a particular set of keystrokes (Contol + Shift + Enter) required to perform mathematical functions on matrices or arrays. Requires determining "footprint" of the result in advance.

Association Analysis A branch of analytics designed to analyze "marketbasket" types of data, typically nominal, and based on counting occurrences.

Assumptions Principles that are inherent and (to a greater or lesser degree) required for a mathematical approach to be valid.

Bagging A modeling technique (**b**ootstrap **agg**regating = bagging) used in classification and regression analysis in which a number of input datasets are sampled with replacement from the original dataset, typically averaging the results from the multiple generated models.

Between Groups A term used in analysis of variance for one component of the partitioned variance (as opposed to within groups) which focuses on the variance differences between the groups.

Bias A systematic difference between the observed and the actual. In a "perfect world" there should be no bias, but there often is and must be measured and accounted for.

Bias-Variance Trade-Off An important consideration in selecting the optimum number of input variables (model complexity) in a predictive model.

Bold Bold terms in the text of this book can be found in this glossary.

Boosting Instead of eliminating outliers or hard-to-fit data points, boosting focuses on them, building a model that formally addresses these data points.

© Springer International Publishing Switzerland 2016
P.J. Fabri, *Measurement and Analysis in Transforming Healthcare Delivery*,
DOI 10.1007/978-3-319-40812-5

Brainstorming A group process that gathers information pertinent to a defined issue or question. Often followed by a selection or prioritization step.

Cause and Effect A critical concept in model building. True "cause and effect" can only be ascertained in a prospective, randomized analysis which isolates the variables that are manipulated. Any retrospective analysis can, at best, provide an inference to causality with varying risk of error.

Centering A technique of making data more homogeneous by subtracting the group mean from each data point in the set.

Central Tendency A measure of "centeredness" accomplished by the mean (mathematical average and parametric), the median (middlemost value and nonparametric), or mode (most frequent occurrence).

Centroid A multidimensional approach to a central tendency of a group of data, as opposed to "medoid."

Chart* A group of functions in Excel that provide menu-driven visualization/graphing capability.

Classification A branch of analytics using computer methods to assign individual "subjects" to classes or groups based on supervised learning.

Clustering A branch of analytics using computer methods to identify potential groupings or clusters based on some measure of distance or similarity, using unsupervised learning.

Coefficient of Determination A simple but powerful measure of the percent of total variance that can be explained by a mathematical model. Known as R-squared.

Collinearity A consideration in a dataset representing the degree of correlation between variables. Also known as multicollinearity.

Computer Software A "package" of computer codes designed and composed to perform defined tasks or functions, often combined in a set of tasks/functions.

Concordance Mathematical measure of agreement, often between two or more raters. More generally, the degree to which "things" agree.

Conditional Formatting* Excel function which allows all cells that share some attribute or property to be visually identified.

Conditional Probability The probability or likelihood of something GIVEN that something else exists or is considered to exist.

Conditioning Variables Dividing a total group into a set of identifiable subgroups, thus allocating the total likelihood into the sum of conditional likelihoods.

Confidence Interval Confidence is based on the standard error of the mean. The confidence interval is typically set at 2 SEM. Confidence interval provides an estimate for how widely a repeat measure of the mean would be expected to vary. See tolerance interval.

Correlation* The degree that variables are mathematically correlated (Pearson's correlation coefficient). In Excel, a function in Analysis Toolpak that creates correlation matrices for multiple variables.

Covariance Matrix A square, triangularly symmetrical matrix, with variances of each variable on the diagonal and covariances otherwise. Represented by Σ.

Covariance* A mathematical "cousin" of correlation, used in many complex mathematical functions and processes. (Correlation is "understandable," but covariance is how to do the math.)

Covariates Many different definitions, so be careful. Could be "big factors" or "groupings" represented as data variables. Could simply be input variables. Could be components of analysis of covariance (ANCOVA).

Cox Proportional Hazard Analysis A model-based technique, based on survival methodology, that determines a family of exponentials, each of which has a linear function as the exponent, used to analyze contributing factors in survival models. Very dependent on assumptions, however.

Cumulative Distribution Function (cdf) A method of describing the cumulative fraction of an ordered (small to large) data set, ranging from 0 to 100%. The cumulative fraction of data points for all values less than a chosen value of x. Mathematically, the cdf is the integral of the pdf.

Curse of Dimensionality A phrase which applies to the bias-variance trade-off. As in "Goldilocks," a model can be too small, too large, or just right.

Data The most basic of inputs, a set of numbers or words, to which meaning, context, analysis, and synthesis can be added.

Data Analysis* The "menu name" in Excel for the Analysis Toolpak.

Database An organized collection of data stored in computer-readable memory. Often a hierarchical and relational collection of "objects."

Dataframes A term used in some software (such as "R") to describe a structured collection of data that contains non-numeric variables, to distinguish it from a true matrix or array.

Dataset The common term used to describe a collection of structured data, often acquired or "queried" from a database, that is then delivered to someone for analysis.

Deduction/Deductive An important concept in logic that finds use in understanding "hypothesis testing." A deduction is an answer to a mathematical or logical proposition that is deterministic (unavoidable). The answer to $2 + 2 =$, for example, is always "4."

Defects The actual number of defects, as for example, the number of complications during a hospitalization. Used in statistical process control.

Defectives The frequency of unacceptable units either as the number per unit time or the proportion. Used in statistical process control.

Degrees of Freedom (df) An important concept in statistics as it represents an "adjusted" measure of sample size. When parameters have been calculated for a set of data, in resampling typically all but one of the entities can take any value, but the last one will already be "determined" by the mean; thus $n-1$ is the most common (but not the only) df.

Dependent A term usually applied to an outcome variable (the dependent variable) as opposed to the input variables (independent variables).

Descriptive Statistics* In Excel, an important method contained in data analysis, which performs a battery of common statistical tests to allow an initial assessment of the data.

Deviations A term often confused with two others, residuals and errors. Deviations are differences between an observed value and some other reference value. An error is a deviation from the true value, while a residual is a deviation from an expected value, often the mean.

Dimensionality A term describing the complexity of a model, often represented by the number of variables (or dimensions) of the input data.

Distance A term describing a measure of how "far" away something is from something else. Proximity (quantitative) and similarity (qualitative) are typical forms of distance measures.

Distributions (of Data) A term describing known (or empirical) frequency curves for a set of data. The most well known (but actually only one of many) is the normal or Gaussian distribution.

Ensemble A term used to describe the combination of a number of different methodological approaches to modeling something, so as to produce a single, representative model.

Epistemology "How we know what we know" or literally the study of knowledge (philosophy). The scientific study is called "epistemics."

Error The difference between a measurement and its true value. See deviations.

Euclidean Distance A form of measuring distance using the sum of squared distances, essentially the hypotenuse or "straight-line": distance. Formally known as the L2 norm. (The sum of the component distances, as in walking on city streets instead of flying like a crow, is the L1 norm or Manhattan distance.)

Failure Mode and Effect Analysis (FMEA) A process originating in engineering and often applied in healthcare settings. It is a forward-looking brainstorming process in which a group of carefully selected subject matter experts are asked to put together a comprehensive list of everything that could possibly go wrong (failure modes) and then assess three attributes (effects) of each: frequency, severity, and undetectability.

Find and Select* A menu command in Excel that includes a number of methods to find, replace, and special variations of find/replace items in a spreadsheet. Very useful for establishing a visual assessment of how many and where in a large spreadsheet.

Hazard Function An important derived measure in survival analysis, the cumulative hazard function is minus the log of the derivative of the survival curve. It can be thought of as the likelihood of surviving given that you have survived to a defined point, mathematically the first derivative of survival divided by survival. The simplest way to think about it is, at a given point, is the risk of failure going to increase, decrease, or stay constant. it is the underlying basis of the Cox proportional hazard analysis.

Heteroscedastic, Heteroscedasticity Literally different dispersion, but commonly unequal variance. Many statistical methods assume constant and equal variance, so heteroscedasticity represents a deviation from the assumptions and needs to be addressed.

Histogram* An Excel method in data analysis for depicting graphically the vertical bar graph of the frequencies of the data.

Home* An Excel menu that contains a number of important analytics functions for spreadsheet use.

Homogeneity of Variances An assumption of many statistical methods, similar in meaning to homoscedasticity, meaning equal shape and size of the variances.

Homoscedastic, Homoscedasticity Literally same dispersions, commonly equal variances.

Hyperspace See multidimensional space.

Hypothesis A statement of belief. In the scientific method, starting with a belief (hypothesis), one creates a null hypothesis (the belief is not true). Statistical tests measure the credibility of the null hypothesis by attempting to reject it, thus accepting the alternate hypothesis or belief. In a designed experiment, the hypothesis (and null) is established before the experiments are conducted and the data are collected; thus the null and the alternate are already defined. In retrospective analytics, a hypothesis (and its null) is generated from the data, requiring a reinterpretation of the p-values of hypothesis testing and rejecting the null.

Hypothesis Testing The underlying probability theory behind statistical tests: a hypothesis is converted to a null hypothesis, and the null tested for possible rejection.

Independent A confusing term, so be careful. In creating models, independent refers to the input variables and dependent to the outcome variable(s). In statistics, independent means not correlated and thus having no covariance. The fact that something is independent in model-building does NOT mean it is independent statistically (and very often isn't!).

Induction, Inductive An important concept in logic that finds use in understanding "hypothesis testing." An induction starts with the answer and considers what the question might have been. For example, if the answer is "4," a possible question might be $2 + 2 - ?$. But there are certainly many other possible questions, so there is a large element of what is likely. This is important in analytics, because only inferences (induction) are possible when considering retrospective data. Once an inference is reached, the next question should be how likely is this to be true.

Information When "data" are given a meaning, they become "information." When "information" is given a context, it becomes "knowledge." When "knowledge" is analyzed, synthesized, and interpreted, it becomes "wisdom."

Input In modeling, the input variables are used to build the model relative to the outcome or output variables.

Insert * There are two important aspects of input in Excel: a drop-down menu and a right click function. The drop-down menu produces a variety of options including Pivot Tables, Charts, Equations, Symbols, and more. The right click function allows a new row or column to be inserted into a spreadsheet with control over what gets moved where.

Instrumental Variables Input variables that quantitatively substitute for one or more unmeasured but important variables in models that infer causality.

Interquartile Range (IQR) A nonparametric assessment of the dispersion of a dataset, conceptually analogous to standard deviation. It is the difference between the values at the 25th percentile and the 75th percentile (first and third quartiles). The IQR is approximately 1 1/3 times the standard deviation if the data are normally distributed.

Jaccard Coefficient A calculated measure of similarity that ignores zero values. Athematically, the ratio of the intersection (and) and the union (or) of two datasets.

Asymmetric Dataset This is a special use of "asymmetric," meaning that the dataset is comprised exclusively of zeroes and ones, binary.

Knowledge A level of understanding after data has been "raised" to information by adding meaning, and "information" has been raised to knowledge, by adding context.

Kurtosis A term used to describe a distribution function that is taller and thinner (leptokurtosis) or shorter and fatter (platykurtosis) than a normal, Gaussian distribution. Kurtosis is the fourth moment of a distribution.

Labels in First Row A common convention in spreadsheets in which the variable names are placed at the top of adjacent columns, all in the top row.

Lead-Time Bias In clinical medicine, lead-time bias refers to an APPARENT change in survival after the introduction of a new diagnostic modality which allows diagnosis at an earlier time or stage of disease.

Length Bias In clinical medicine, length bias (or length-time bias) refers to a type of selection bias in which a new diagnostic modality unknowingly selects out that is not only "earlier" but also "less aggressive," leading to a possible misinterpretation of survival.

Likelihood A close cousin of probability. Likelihood refers to relative frequency of occurrence based on empirical observation from data, whereas probability is defined scientifically. However, the two terms are often used interchangeably.

Logistic In statistics, the logistic (which can be thought of as the inverse of the logit—see logit) is $1/(1+e^{-x})$, which is a probability.

Logit See logistic. In statistics the logit is $\log(x/(1-x))$ which is" log-odds."

Log-Rank In survival analysis, the log-rank test compares two survival curves.

Machine Learning A term used to describe mathematical models generated by high-speed computers from large datasets.

Mahalanobis Distance A multidimensional analog of Euclidean distance, standardized by the covariance matrix.

Manhattan Distance A distance measure, also known as L1 or city-block distance, because of how one would walk from point to point on city streets.

Marginal Plot A visualization method in which a scatterplot has histograms on the top and right side, showing the corresponding distributions.

Market-Basket A term applied to association analysis, used to describe a collection of nominal objects, as in a shopping basket at a market.

Matrix A two-dimensional array that contains only numeric entries.

Matrix Mathematics See Array Function. A set of rules for performing mathematical manipulations of matrices: addition/subtraction, multiplication, inversion.

Maximum The largest entity in a set of data, or the peak value in a function at which point the slope is zero (a horizontal line).

Mean The mathematical average of a set of numbers. A parametric measure of central tendency, which is the first moment of a distribution.

Mean Squared Error (MSE) Equivalent to "variance," the MSE is a specific sum of squared residuals divided by the corresponding df (degrees of freedom).

Median The middlemost of a set of numbers. A nonparametric measure of central tendency.

Medoid See centroid. A medoid is an actual data point closest to the central tendency of a set of data, especially a cluster.

Metrics Standardized method of measuring or quantitating an entity.

Middleware Computer software whose primary function is to bridge between two other software packages (often a popular package and a difficult package), or which provides functions not available in the operating system.

Minimum The smallest value in a dataset of the lowest point in a distribution with a slope of zero (horizontal line). See maximum.

Missing Values Many software methods only work when there is a value for every cell. Empty cells are called "missing values." Typically missing values need to be addressed.

Mode The "softest" measure of central tendency, the mode is the most likely value in a unimodal (one peak) distribution. It is useful in determining a triangular distribution.

Model Specifically, a replica of something, usually simplified. In analytics, a mathematical equation that describes a dataset or predicts an outcome. The model is typically an "imperfect" replica, with varying degrees of uncertainty and error.

Modeling The process of creating a mathematical model from a dataset.

Modified Delphi Process A survey-based method of prioritizing a list generated by brainstorming, which typically converges to a consensus. See nominal group process.

Most Likelihood Estimation (MLE) A concept and associated group of statistical methods that use maximization methods to optimize the parameters/coefficients in a model.

Multicollinearity See collinearity. The presence of correlation in a multidimensional dataset.

Multidimensional Space Although only one-, two-, and three-dimensional space can readily be "visualized," any number of independent variables can be interpreted as a multidimensional space, also known as hyperspace.

Multiple Regression A form of regression which utilizes more than one input variable. While most commonly linear, transformed data can produce nonlinear regressions.

New Worksheet An Excel workbook can hold as many worksheets as the computer memory will allow. A new worksheet can be created by right-clicking an existing worksheet tab at the bottom of an Excel worksheet and clicking on insert:new worksheet.

Nominal One of the four types of variables (nominal, ordinal, interval, ratio) comprising "words" that have a sense of order but no actual quantitative metric.

Nominal Group Process A structured brainstorming methodology, designed to provide a safe environment to develop comprehensive lists of possible events.

Nominal Attributes Qualitative attributes of an entity, object, or variable.

Nonhomogeneous When applied to a distribution, nonhomogeneous describes one of a number of forms of unequal variance across the data.

Normal Distribution Synonym for a Gaussian (bell-shaped) distribution, characterized by the parameters of mean and standard deviation. While historically called "normal" because of a belief that it was widely correct, it is now known that many entities should be described by other types of distribution: exponential for time-based data, gamma for waiting times, Weibull for failure rates, and log-normal for many biochemical measurements.

Null Hypothesis The cornerstone of the scientific method consisting of the logical process of stating a hypothesis in the negative (null hypothesis) and using statistical methods to demonstrate that this belief is unlikely to be true.

Objective Function The "answer" that is maximized or minimized in an optimization process.

Objects In computer terminology, simple data are usually a number or a word. But advanced computer languages can actually manipulate "objects," much more complex than a number or word. An object is an entity (it actually exists), which has defined properties and actions. Most simply, an object is something in a computer that can be cut and pasted.

Odds A way to think about and use probability mathematically. The ratio of the probability of yes divided by the probability of no, often symbolized as $x/(1-x)$.

Optimization A mathematical process, usually based on linear programming or gradient ascent methods, for determining the optimum set of values to maximize or minimize an objective function.

Options* In Excel, a menu command that displays options. Useful for finding and installing "add-ins" as well as other optional functions.

Ordinal One of the four types of variables (nominal, ordinal, interval, ratio) comprising "words" that have a sense of order but no actual quantitative metric.

Outcome A variable used as the result of a model, as in actual outcome or expected outcome. Usually designated as y (actual) or $\hat{y}$ (expected).

Outlier A value that is so removed from the central tendency or expected value so as to suspect that it came from somewhere else.

Overdiagnosis Bias A term used in clinical medicine and epidemiology, especially when a new diagnostic method (lab or imaging) identifies many more instances than have been clinically apparent.

Overfitting A term applied to creating a predictive model with more input variables than actually required, which makes the model superficially look better but actually perform worse.

$p < 0.05$ The typical default in hypothesis testing. Often misinterpreted to mean "important" or "useful," $p < 0.05$ simply means how willing am I to be wrong.

Paired A specific example of "matching," pairing occurs when separate measurements are obtained IN THE SAME SUBJECT, so that all other attributes remain the same (except treatment or time). Analysis is then based on the difference in the measurements with the strong assumption that everything else is the same.

Parameters Attributes of a model-based measurement. Once calculated, the parameters replace the actual data, so if the model is wrong (e.g., normality), so is the analysis.

Partitioning When applied to analysis of variance, partitioning means allocating the total variance into meaningful subsets and then comparing them.

Paste Special* In Excel, an area (now an object!) that is copied can be pasted in a number of ways, which can be found by hovering over Paste or by clicking Paste Special. These variations on Paste are worth knowing.

Pivot Table In Excel, a menu-driven approach to "slicing and dicing" a set of data to enhance understanding and to examine aggregations of the data.

Platykurtosis/Platykurtotic A symmetrical distribution, resembling a normal distribution, but flatter and wider, thus not actually "normally distributed."

Precision The repeatability of a measurement. Even if it is inaccurate, it can be precise. This is equivalent to valid but not reliable.

Predictive Models In machine learning, a model based on using known outcomes to develop the ability to predict new input observations (yet without outcomes).

Predictive Relationship In causality analysis, when there is correlation it is tempting to say "predictive." A truly predictive relationship exists when the correlation is so high that the outcome is very likely. Typically this is an R-squared of at least 90%.

Predictive Value of a Negative Test (PVN or NPV) A concept related "conditionally" to specificity and of more interest to clinicians. Specificity applies to a measurement (e.g., lab test) in someone who is already known NOT to have a disease. NPV applies to the likelihood of NO DISEASE in a subject with a normal test result.

Predictive Value of a Positive Test (PVP or PPV) A concept related "conditionally" to sensitivity and of more interest to clinicians. Sensitivity applies to a measurement (e.g., lab test) in some who is already known TO HAVE A DISEASE. PPV applies to the likelihood of disease actually present when a subject has an abnormal test result.

Probability A measure of how likely something is to occur (e.g., flipping heads) in a situation where that likelihood is actually known by theory or principle.

Probability and Statistics A "bucket" term for anything and everything having to do with probability and statistics, but often used to name an education course.

Probability Distribution Function (pdf) A mathematical expression of the probability of an event as a function of an input (x). The best understood pdf is the normal or Gaussian curve, but that is only one of a large number of pdfs. The pdf is the first derivative of the cdf.

Process A set of interconnected steps that lead to a product or outcome.

Projection A corresponding value on one of a set of perpendicular axes. "Dropping a perpendicular" produces a projection on that axis.

Propensity Score A mathematical approach to creating comparable groups in retrospective data, to more closely approximate unbiased sampling.

Proximity A distance measure (see similarity) which is quantitative.

Pseudoreplication An important distinction from true replication. Pseudoreplication consists of making multiple measurements OF THE SAME ENTITY, while true replication consists of a set of identical but individual "experiments." Weighing ten sets of ten pennies is replication; weighing one set of ten pennies ten times is pseudoreplication. This is important because pseudoreplication does not increase "n," sample size.

Quantile (QQ) Plots A visualization method that compares the quantiles of a first distribution with those of a second, or of one variable dimension with a second. Agreement should give a straight plot.

Random Sampling A process of selecting subjects based on an actual random number table or software method. More than just the "appearance" of randomness.

Range* The difference between the maximum and minimum in a dataset. A very "rough" measure of dispersion.

Rank* An Excel command that determines the position of a value in the ordered arrangement of a dataset, e.g., 7th smallest.

Ratio One of the four types of variables (nominal, ordinal, interval, ratio) comprising true quantities that have a zero value and which can undergo all mathematical manipulations.

Regression A mathematical or statistical method that determines the relationship of an outcome to one or more input variables "as a function of…."

Regression in Excel* Excel has three programmed methods for performing regression: "=LINEST," "Regression" in Data Analysis, and "f(x)" in scatterplot. $f(x)$ is the simplest, regression is the most comprehensive, and =LINEST is the most useful from a programming/calculation perspective.

Reliability A measure of the reproducibility of a measurement, which could be very incorrect but repeatable. See validity.

Remove Duplicates* An Excel command that identifies and removes entities in a column that are exactly the same.

Repeated Measures An important concept in statistics which represents measuring the same attribute IN THE SAME SUBJECT after an intervention or the passage of time, typically including a control. The assumption is that since it is the same subject, all other aspects remain the same. Analysis of "repeated measures" is different from other serial assessments.

Replication See pseudoreplication. True replication requires independent "experiments," rather than measuring the same entity multiple times.

Residual/Residuals The difference between the actual value and the expected value. Most of modern statistics are based on measuring and analyzing residuals. Graphic visualization of residuals is very useful in assessing the fit of assumed distributions.

Response Surface A visualization method for an outcome variable (the response) as a function of input variables. The resulting "surface" created is the response surface.

Retrospective Analysis The process of analyzing data AFTER the data were collected, especially historical data. Typically, the data were not collected for the current purpose.

R-Squared The coefficient of determination, which is actually the square of the correlation coefficient in 2D. R-squared can be generalized to higher dimensions, with adjustment.

Sample A finite number of observations gathered either systematically or randomly from a presumed or theoretical larger population.

Sample Size: What is Small Sample size, the number of observations in a set of measurements, must be assessed in interpreting statistics. When the sample size is smaller than 30, unusual things are more likely to occur, so $n < 30$ is considered "small." This behavior led to the development of the Student t-test for small samples. This concern is much less for samples $30 < n < 100$, and all but eliminated for $n > 100$.

Scientific Method A structured approach to experimentation in which a tentative hypothesis (of a difference) is converted to a null hypothesis (no difference), and a designed experiment conducted after establishing the statistics to be performed. If the null is unlikely, it is rejected and the alternate hypothesis accepted (without actually testing it).

Similarity A measure of "distance" for non-quantifiable entities. There are many definitions of similarity, best distinguished from the easier concept, dissimilarity.

Simple Matching Coefficient A quantitation of degree of agreement, typically of binary variables, which also includes zero values (see Jaccard coefficient).

Skewness* A measure of asymmetry of a distribution, corresponding to a "directional tail," such as tail-to-the-right. Skewness is the "third moment" of a distribution.

Software The common-usage term to describe a set of computer programs in a package, usually commercially available, organized around a "theme," such as "statistical software."

Sort* An Excel command in the "Data" menu, which sorts a dataset based on selected variable(s), in a hierarchical structure.

Stacking A term used in statistical software that takes similar and corresponding columns of data and assembles them "vertically" into a single column plus an identifier column.

Standard Deviation* A measure of dispersion, representing the square root of the variance. A standard deviation can be calculated for any set of data, but only has a clear meaning if the distribution is normal, Gaussian.

Standard Error A measure of dispersion of the mean result of a sample or experiment, a value smaller than the standard deviation (which applies to dispersion of individual measurements). The SEM is mathematically equal to the standard deviation divided by the square root of "n."

Standard Errors The number of standard errors corresponds to the "confidence interval" for a measurement. Typically two standard errors, which represent the 95th percentile of confidence, are used. It establishes how widely the average of an independent sample from the same population would be expected to vary.

Standardizing A structured approach to creating a "unit value" for a measure, achieved by subtracting the mean and then dividing by the standard deviation. While it can be applied to any set of data, it is most easily understood when the data are normally distributed.

Statistical Process Control (SPC) A structured method which uses both mathematics and graphics to assess the outcome/product of a process, for example in manufacturing. It establishes control limits (typically 3SD) that can identify an extreme outlier and justify "stopping the line."

Stochastic When related to a variable means that it is "random." Implicit is the concept of random variation over time.

Subject Matter Experts (SMEs) SMEs are important in providing less biased interpretation or context of data/observations.

Sum of Residuals Literally the sum of a set of deviations from the mean. Since they are all referenced against the mean, the sum of residuals should be zero. For this reason, either the absolute value or the square is used.

Sum of Squared Residuals An aggregate measure of total variability which, when divided by adjusted sample size, yields the variance or mean square error.

Sum of Squares While this may apply to a sum of products, it usually is the short form of **sum of squared residuals**.

Summary Statistics Statistical software typically has some function to generate a set of summary statistics. In Excel, this is called descriptive statistics.

Sumproduct * An Excel command that generates the sum of the individual products of corresponding elements in two columns or rows of data of equal length. When applied to the same set, this yields the sum of squares.

Supervised A type of machine learning in which a predictive model is generated using a known and measured set of outcomes to "train" the model.

Supervised Learning Short for supervised machine learning. See supervised and machine learning.

Survival Function The mathematical formulation of the rate of survival over time; the percentage of individuals still alive at the end of a time interval who were alive at the beginning of the interval.

Survival Methods A group of methods used to analyze survival data in clinical medicine and epidemiology.

Survival See survival function.

System A set of interrelated processes that share a common goal, but not a specific product or outcome. See process.

Test Application of a formal analysis to address a question or hypothesis.

Text-to-Columns* An Excel menu command (Home) that partitions a column of data into two or more columns based on either width or a specified "separating variable," often a comma.

Time Series Both a series of data based on time and an approach to periodicity analysis, using some mathematical function to mimic the periodicity, e.g., Fourier analysis.

Tolerance Interval Similar to confidence interval but based on the standard deviation, typically 2 or 3 SD. The tolerance interval is an estimate of how widely an individual measurement would be expected to vary.

Total Variance In ANOVA, regression, and other methods, the total sum of squared residuals divided by the df. The total SSR is then partitioned into logical components and divided by the respective df to produce partitioned MSE.

Transform A mathematical function that converts a set of data into another form, e.g., taking the logarithm of time-measured data.

Transpose Term used to describe flipping a matrix in which rows become columns and vice versa.

Triangular Distribution A relatively simple approach for creating a distribution from empiric data utilizing only the smallest, largest, and most frequent values.

T-Test A robust statistical test that evaluates the likelihood of a distance between two means relative to an expression of the standard error calculated from the data; a difference of more than 2 SEM suggests that the null hypothesis of no difference should be rejected.

T-Test Paired Two Sample for Means* In Excel, a command in data analysis used to perform a *t*-test on two columns of data that can appropriately be paired.

T-Test-Two-Sample Assuming Equal Variance* A type of *t*-test which compares two independent columns of data which have been shown to have roughly equal variance measures.

T-Test-Two-Sample Assuming Unequal Variance A type of *t*-test which compares two independent columns of data which have been shown to have unequal variances.

Two-Step Regression An approach to data analysis using regression in which an initial step to transform the data using regression has been performed. See instrumental variable.

Unbalanced Data Data in which there is a marked difference in size between groups. Statistical models rely, to a greater or lesser extent, on equal group sizes and deviation can lead to incorrect conclusions.

Unsupervised See unsupervised learning.

Unsupervised Learning A form of machine learning which does not have an outcome or alternatively ignores the outcome for purposes of identifying "structure" in the dataset, e.g., clustering.

Validation The process of confirming the usefulness of a predictive model by testing the model on a new set of data which were not used in creating the model.

Validity Another word for accuracy, often used in association with reliability.

Values only* An option available in Past Special (Excel) which removes underlying formulas and pastes the data in the same exact form as the original.

Variability A broad term that describes the level of uncertainty or stochasticity of a variable or dataset.

Variance A measure of dispersion based on the sum of squared residuals (SSR), which results in units different from the original data, synonymous with mean squared error. Variance is the second moment of a distribution.

Vector A measurement which has both quantity and direction. However, any data point in a dimensional space can be represented as a vector from the origin of the coordinate axes to the point. Therefore a vector can be considered to be a collection of similar entities, thus a column of data or a row of data in a structured spreadsheet.

Visualization A technique for graphically demonstrating relationships contained within data.

Western Electric Rules A set of structured rules for using statistical process control which define specific reasons to "stop the line" and analyze the process.

Wisdom Wisdom is reached by providing meaning, context, and synthesis/analysis to data.

Within Groups A term describing a partition of variance that allows an assessment or comparison of differences between more than two groups.

Z-Test A generalizable equivalent of a t-test, accomplished by standardizing the difference between two variables, used when sample size is >30.

Bibliography

These references will provide a background for the concepts addressed in this book. Each reference was selected because it is understandable, well documented, and has a comprehensive bibliography of its own.

Anscombe FJ. Graphs in statistical analysis. Am Stat. 1973;27(1):17–21.

Askin RG, Standridge CR. Modeling and analysis of manufacturing systems. New York: Wiley; 1993.

Bailar JC, Hoaglin DC. Medical uses of statistics. New York: John Wiley & Sons; 2012.

Benneyan J, Lloyd R, Plsek P. Statistical process control as a tool for research and healthcare improvement. Qual Saf Health Care. 2003;12(6):458–64.

Berthold M, Hand DJ. Intelligent data analysis: an introduction. 2 rev. and extended edth ed. New York: Springer; 2003.

Bewick V, Cheek L, Ball J. Statistics review 12: survival analysis. Crit Care. 2004;8:389–94.

Bower JA. Statistical methods for food science: introductory procedures for the food practitioner. Chichester: Wiley-Blackwell; 2009.

Crawley MJ. Statistical computing: an introduction to data analysis using S-Plus. Chichester: Wiley; 2002.

Crawley MJ. Statistics: an introduction using R. 2nd ed. Hoboken: Wiley; 2014.

Crawley MJ. The R book. 2nd ed. Chichester: Wiley; 2013.

Dalgaard P. SpringerLink. Introductory statistics with R. 2nd ed. New York: Springer; 2008.

Dretzke BJ. Statistics with Microsoft Excel. 4th ed. Upper Saddle River: Prentice Hall; 2009.

Hamel LH. Knowledge discovery with support vector machines, vol. 3. New York: John Wiley & Sons; 2011.

Hand DJ, Mannila H, Smyth P. Principles of data mining. Cambridge, MA: MIT Press; 2001.

Hand DJ. Statistics and the Theory of Measurement. J R Stat Soc Ser A. 1996;150(3):445–92.

Hand DJ. The improbability principle: why coincidences, miracles, and rare events happen every day. 1st ed. New York: Scientific American/Farrar, Straus and Giroux; 2014.

Hastie T, Friedman JH, Tibshirani R. The elements of statistical learning: data mining, inference, and prediction. 2, corrected 7 printing edth ed. New York: Springer; 2009.

Hastie T, James G, Tibshirani R, Witten D. An introduction to statistical learning: with applications in R. New York: Springer; 2013.

© Springer International Publishing Switzerland 2016   175

P.J. Fabri, *Measurement and Analysis in Transforming Healthcare Delivery*,
DOI 10.1007/978-3-319-40812-5

Heiberger RM, Holland B. Statistical analysis and data display: an intermediate course with examples in S-plus, R, and SAS. New York: Springer Science + Business Media; 2004.

Heiberger RM, Neuwirth E. SpringerLink. R through Excel a spreadsheet interface for statistics, data analysis, and graphics. New York: Springer; 2009.

Hess KR. Graphical methods for assessing violations of the proportional hazards assumption in Cox regression. Stat Med. 1995;14(15):1707–23.

Imai M. Kaizen (Ky'zen), the key to Japan's competitive success. 1st ed. New York: Random House Business Division; 1986.

Klein J, Rizzo J, Zhang M, Keiding N. MINI-REVIEW-Statistical methods for the analysis and presentation of the results of bone marrow transplants. Part I: unadjusted analysis. Bone Marrow Transplant. 2001;28(10):909–16.

Kutner MH, Nachtsheim C, Neter J. Applied linear regression models. 4th ed. New York: McGraw-Hill; 2004.

McDermott RE, Mikulak RJ, Beauregard MR. The basics of FMEA. 2nd ed. New York: Productivity Press; 2009.

McGrayne SB. The theory that would not die: how Bayes' rule cracked the enigma code, hunted down Russian submarines, & emerged triumphant from two centuries of controversy. New Haven, CT: Yale University Press; 2011.

Montgomery DC. Introduction to statistical quality control. 7th ed. Hoboken, NJ: Wiley; 2013.

Morgan SL, Winship C. Counterfactuals and causal inference: methods and principles for social research. New York: Cambridge University Press; 2007.

Newton I. Minitab Cookbook. Birmingham: Packt Publishing; 2014.

Pace L. Beginning R, an introduction to statistical programming. New York: Apress; 2012. Distributed to the book trade worldwide by Springer Science + Business Media.

Quirk TJ, Horton H, Quirk M. Excel 2010 for biological and life sciences statistics a guide to solving practical problems. New York, NY: Springer; 2013.

Quirk TJ, Cummings S. Excel 2010 for health services management statistics: a guide to solving practical problems. Cham: Springer; 2014.

Schmuller J. Statistical analysis with Excel for dummies. 2nd ed. John Wiley & Sons, Inc: Hoboken; 2009.

Schumacker RE, Tomek S. Understanding statistics using R. New York, NY: Springer; 2013.

Shumway RH, Stoffer DS. Time series analysis and its applications: with R examples. New York: Springer Science & Business Media; 2010.

Spector P. SpringerLink. Data manipulation with R. New York: Springer Verlag; 2008.

Steinwart I, Christmann A. SpringerLink. Support vector machines. 1st ed. New York: Springer; 2008.

Stigler SM. Statistics on the table: the history of statistical concepts and methods. Cambridge, MA: Harvard University Press; 1999.

Taleb N. The black swan: the impact of the highly improbable. 1st ed. New York: Random House; 2007.

Tan H. Knowledge discovery and data mining. New York: Springer; 2012.

Tan PN, Steinbach M, Kumar V. Introduction to data mining. Boston: Pearson-Addison Wesley; 2006.

Teetor P, Loukides MK. R cookbook. 1st ed. Beijing: O'Reilly; 2011.

Tufte ER. The visual display of quantitative information. 2nd ed. Cheshire, CT: Graphics Press; 2001.

Veney JE, Kros JF, Rosenthal DA. Statistics for health care professionals working with Excel. 2nd ed. San Francisco: Jossey-Bass; 2009.

Index

A
Actuarial survival, 131, 134, 135
Advanced Analytical Software, 21
"Affine" function, 82
Akaike Information Criterion (AIC), 96
Alternate hypothesis, 88
Analysis of variance (ANOVA)
    complex ANOVA, 41
    degrees of freedom (df), 41
    description, 41
    forms, Data Analysis, 41
    "F-test", 41
    replication and pseudo-replication, 43
    Single Factor, 42
Analytics, 4, 7, 8
Arrays, 83
Association analysis, 6
    association rule, 123
    confidence, 123
    frequent itemsets, 122, 123
    hospital-level data, 122
    infrequent itemsets, 125
    itemset, 123
    nominal variables, 124
    preoperative laboratory test, 122
    sparse dataset, 123
    support, 123
    transactions, 121
    transaction-type dataset, 124
Attribute charts, 148

B
Bayes' theorem, 89, 144
Bayesian Information Criterion (BIC), 96

Bias, 70
Bias-variance trade-off, 81, 84–85
Bootstrap analysis, 96
Bradford-Hill criteria, 141

C
Cause and effect, 9
    errors, hypothesis testing, 142, 143
    p-Values, 142
    sensitivity and specificity,
        143–144
    Simpson's paradox, 140, 141
Censoring, survival analysis, 133
Centering, 73
Clustering, 7
    density-based, 126, 127
    description, 125
    fuzzy clustering, 126
    hierarchical clustering, 126
    "k" clusters, 126
    K-means, 126
    K-nearest-neighbor (knn) clustering, 126
    model-based clustering, 129
    multidimensional data, 125
    validation, 127–129
Comprehensive R Archive Network (CRAN),
    56, 57
Conditional probability, 89
Continuous quality improvement, 3
Cox proportional hazard model, 131,
    134, 136
Cross-validation, 95
Cumulative distribution function (cdf), 65
Curse of dimensionality, 84

© Springer International Publishing Switzerland 2016
P.J. Fabri, *Measurement and Analysis in Transforming Healthcare Delivery*,
DOI 10.1007/978-3-319-40812-5

Printed in the United States
By Bookmasters